GASTRIC BYPASS COOKBOOK

A comprehensive guide with 150+ Nutrient-rich recipes to support healing and healthy eating post-gastric bypass surgery

TERESA MILLER

COPYRIGHT ©

All rights reserved.

No part of this book may be reproduced in any form or by any electronic or mechanical means, including information storage and retrieval systems, without permission in writing from the publisher, except by a reviewer who may quote brief passages in a review.

The information contained in this book is based on the author's research and experience. While the author has made every effort to provide accurate and up-to-date information, errors and omissions may occur. The author and publisher assume no responsibility for any errors or omissions or for any actions taken based on the information contained in this book.

The information contained in this book is provided "as is," without warranty of any kind, express or implied, including but not limited to the warranties of merchantability, fitness for a particular purpose, or non-infringement. In no event shall the author or publisher be liable for any claim, damages, or other liability, whether in an action of contract, tort, or otherwise, arising from, out of, or in connection with the book or the use or other dealings in the book.

TABLE OF CONTENTS

CONCLUSION --234

INTRODUCTION

Gastric bypass surgery stands as a transformative journey toward a healthier and more fulfilling life for many individuals struggling with obesity and related health complications. More than just a surgical procedure, it signifies a pivotal step in reshaping both body and lifestyle, offering a renewed chance at overall wellness.

Gastric bypass surgery, a type of bariatric surgery, involves the alteration of the digestive system to aid in weight loss and promote healthier living. This surgical intervention works by reducing the size of the stomach and rerouting a portion of the small intestine, thereby altering the digestive process. Through this restructuring, it limits the amount of food one can consume and alters the absorption of nutrients, fostering weight loss and aiding in the management of obesity-related health issues.

The primary goal of gastric bypass surgery extends beyond mere weight loss. It aims to provide a sustainable solution for individuals battling severe obesity, particularly those for whom traditional weight loss methods have proven ineffective. Beyond shedding excess pounds, this surgery often leads to significant improvements in associated health conditions, such as type 2 diabetes, high blood pressure, sleep apnea, and joint pain.

The potential benefits of gastric bypass surgery encompass not only physical changes but also remarkable improvements in overall quality of life. Many patients experience increased energy levels, enhanced mobility, improved self-esteem, and a reduced dependence on medications for chronic conditions.

Before undergoing gastric bypass surgery, individuals are typically required to adhere to a prescribed diet and lifestyle modifications. This preparatory phase often involves dietary restrictions, behavioral changes, and consultations with healthcare professionals to ensure optimal health and readiness for the procedure. This pre-surgery diet aids in reducing liver size, making the surgery safer and more effective.

Post-surgery, the dietary landscape undergoes a significant shift. Patients are introduced to carefully curated meal plans that emphasize smaller portions, nutrient-dense foods, and gradual progression from liquid to solid foods. The focus lies in adapting to a new way of eating, maintaining proper nutrition, and establishing healthy eating habits to support weight loss and overall well-being.

Gastric bypass surgery serves as a beacon of hope for individuals battling obesity, offering a chance at a healthier, more fulfilling life. This transformative journey is not merely about physical changes but also encompasses emotional and lifestyle transformations. Understanding the surgery, its purpose, and the pivotal role of diet before and after the procedure lays the groundwork for a successful and sustainable path toward long-term health and wellness.

CHAPTER ONE

WHAT IS GASTRIC BYPASS SURGERY?

Gastric bypass surgery, also known as Roux-en-Y gastric bypass, is a type of weight-loss surgery or bariatric surgery performed on individuals who are severely obese and have been unsuccessful in achieving weight loss through conventional methods like diet and exercise.

The surgery involves making changes to the digestive system to help individuals lose weight by restricting food intake and, to some extent, reducing the body's ability to absorb nutrients. Here's an overview of the procedure:

How Gastric Bypass Surgery Works:

• Stomach Size Reduction: The surgeon creates a smaller stomach pouch by dividing the top part of the stomach from the rest. This pouch is about the size of a walnut and can hold only a small amount of food (approximately one ounce or 30 milliliters).

• Altering Digestive Pathway: The small intestine is then rearranged. The surgeon attaches the lower part of the small intestine directly to the small stomach pouch. This bypasses a section of the small intestine, limiting the absorption of calories and nutrients.

Considerations and Risks:

While gastric bypass surgery can be highly effective in aiding weight loss and improving health, it's not without risks or potential complications. These may include:

• Surgical risks such as infection, bleeding, or adverse reactions to anesthesia.

• Nutritional deficiencies due to reduced nutrient absorption.

• Dumping syndrome, causing nausea, vomiting, weakness, and other symptoms after eating certain foods high in sugar or fat.

• Changes in bowel habits or the risk of developing gallstones.

Eligibility and Consultation:

Candidates for gastric bypass surgery usually undergo a comprehensive evaluation by a healthcare team, including a surgeon, dietitian, psychologist, and other specialists, to determine if they meet the criteria and understand the risks and lifestyle changes required before and after surgery.

Overall, gastric bypass surgery is a significant step for individuals severely affected by obesity, aiming to facilitate weight loss and improve overall health and quality of life. However, it's crucial to discuss all options, potential risks, and expected outcomes thoroughly with healthcare professionals before deciding on this surgical intervention.

THE PURPOSE OF GASTRIC BYPASS SURGERY

The primary purpose of gastric bypass surgery, also known as Roux-en-Y gastric bypass, is to aid in significant weight loss for individuals who are severely obese and have struggled to lose weight through conventional methods such as diet and exercise. However, the surgery offers more than just weight reduction; it aims to address various health concerns associated with obesity while promoting a healthier lifestyle.

Key Purposes of Gastric Bypass Surgery:

• Weight Loss: Gastric bypass surgery is primarily performed to help individuals achieve substantial and sustained weight loss. By altering the digestive system, the surgery restricts the amount of food a person can eat and limits the absorption of calories and nutrients, leading to weight loss.

• Treatment of Obesity-Related Health Conditions: Beyond weight reduction, gastric bypass surgery often leads to improvements or even resolution of obesity-related health issues. These may include:

• Type 2 Diabetes: Many individuals experience significant improvements in insulin sensitivity or even complete remission of type 2 diabetes following surgery.

• Hypertension (High Blood Pressure): Weight loss after gastric bypass can help reduce blood pressure, reducing the risk of heart disease and stroke.

• Sleep Apnea: Improvement or resolution of sleep apnea is frequently observed after substantial weight loss post-surgery.

• Joint Pain and Mobility Issues: Reduced body weight can alleviate stress on joints, resulting in decreased pain and improved mobility.

• Enhanced Quality of Life: The surgery often brings about lifestyle improvements and an increased sense of well-being for individuals. This may include increased energy levels, improved self-esteem, and a reduced reliance on medications for obesity-related conditions.

Considerations and Long-Term Goals:

• Sustainable Weight Loss: Gastric bypass surgery is not a quick fix but a tool that, combined with lifestyle changes, can help individuals achieve long-term weight loss.

• Behavioral and Dietary Changes: To maximize the benefits of the surgery, patients must commit to significant lifestyle changes, including dietary modifications, regular exercise, and behavioral adjustments.

• Healthier Living: The surgery serves as a catalyst for individuals to adopt healthier habits, encouraging a balanced diet and increased physical activity to maintain weight loss and overall well-being.

Gastric bypass surgery serves as a crucial intervention for individuals battling severe obesity, aiming to promote weight loss, improve overall health, and enhance quality of life. However, it requires dedication, commitment to long-term lifestyle changes, and ongoing support from healthcare professionals to achieve sustained success and well-being after the surgery.

Gastric bypass surgery, a type of bariatric surgery, offers several potential benefits for individuals struggling with severe obesity and related health conditions. Here are some key benefits associated with gastric bypass surgery:

1. Substantial and Sustained Weight Loss:

• Significant Weight Reduction: Gastric bypass surgery helps individuals achieve substantial weight loss, typically in the range of 60% to 80% of excess body weight within the first year or two after the procedure.

• Long-Term Maintenance: Many patients experience sustained weight loss over several years following surgery, provided they adhere to dietary and lifestyle changes recommended by healthcare professionals.

2. Improvement or Resolution of Obesity-Related Health Conditions:

• Type 2 Diabetes Improvement or Remission: A significant number of individuals with type 2 diabetes see improvements in blood sugar control post-surgery. Some even experience complete remission of diabetes.

• Reduction in Hypertension (High Blood Pressure): Weight loss following gastric bypass surgery often leads to reduced blood pressure levels, decreasing the risk of cardiovascular complications.

• Improved Cardiovascular Health: The surgery may result in decreased cholesterol levels, improved heart function, and a reduced risk of heart disease and stroke.

• Relief from Sleep Apnea: Many patients experience improvements or complete resolution of sleep apnea symptoms due to weight loss, leading to better sleep quality and reduced daytime fatigue.

3. Enhanced Quality of Life and Well-Being:

• Increased Mobility: Weight loss alleviates stress on joints, reducing joint pain and enhancing mobility and physical activity.

• Improved Mental Health: Patients often report enhanced mood, self-esteem, and overall well-being after significant weight loss, leading to improved mental health.

• Reduced Medication Dependency: Individuals may experience reduced reliance on medications for obesity-related health conditions after successful weight loss, leading to a better quality of life.

4. Metabolic and Hormonal Changes:

• Changes in Hormone Levels: Gastric bypass surgery can lead to changes in gut hormones that regulate appetite and metabolism, contributing to reduced hunger and increased feelings of fullness.

• Improvement in Insulin Sensitivity: The surgery may improve insulin sensitivity and glucose metabolism, leading to better blood sugar control in individuals with diabetes.

Considerations:

It's important to note that while gastric bypass surgery offers significant benefits, it also requires commitment to long-term lifestyle changes, including dietary modifications, regular exercise, and ongoing medical follow-ups. Patients need to work closely with healthcare professionals to maximize the benefits of the surgery and maintain a healthy weight and lifestyle post-surgery. Additionally, there are potential risks and complications associated with the procedure that should be discussed thoroughly with a healthcare provider before making a decision.

THE DIFFERENT TYPES OF GASTRIC BYPASS SURGERIES

Gastric bypass surgery is a type of weight-loss surgery that involves altering the digestive system to assist in weight reduction. There are different types of gastric bypass surgeries, each with its variations in how they reroute the digestive tract. The most common types include:

1. Roux-en-Y Gastric Bypass (RYGB):

Roux-en-Y gastric bypass is the most frequently performed gastric bypass surgery. It involves creating a small stomach pouch by stapling the upper part of the stomach to create a pouch that can hold about an ounce of food. The small intestine is then cut and attached to this small stomach pouch, bypassing the lower part of the stomach and the upper portion of the small intestine.

2. Mini-Gastric Bypass (MGB):

Mini-gastric bypass is a simpler and faster procedure compared to the traditional Roux-en-Y gastric bypass. It involves creating a longer and narrower stomach pouch and connecting it to a loop of the small intestine, allowing food to bypass a portion of the small intestine.

3. Biliopancreatic Diversion with Duodenal Switch (BPD-DS):

Biliopancreatic diversion with duodenal switch is a complex surgery that involves two steps. The first step is similar to sleeve gastrectomy, where a portion of the stomach is removed to create a smaller stomach pouch. The second step involves rerouting the intestines to create two pathways — one for food and one for digestive juices — to reduce calorie absorption.

4. Loop Gastric Bypass (SADI-S):

Loop gastric bypass, also known as Single-Anastomosis Duodenal-Ileal Bypass with Sleeve Gastrectomy (SADI-S), is a modification of the traditional gastric bypass procedure. It involves a sleeve gastrectomy to create a smaller stomach pouch and rerouting the small intestine into two limbs, allowing food to bypass a portion of the small intestine.

Considerations:

Each type of gastric bypass surgery has its advantages, considerations, and potential risks. The choice of procedure depends on factors such as the patient's overall health, BMI (Body Mass Index), and individual medical considerations. It's crucial to discuss the available options thoroughly with a healthcare provider to determine the most suitable approach for achieving weight loss goals while considering potential risks and long-term implications.

THE PROCESS, RISKS, RECOVERY TIME, AND POTENTIAL COMPLICATIONS OF ROUX-EN-Y GASTRIC BYPASS.

Roux-en-Y Gastric Bypass (RYGB) is a common type of weight-loss surgery that involves creating a smaller stomach pouch and rerouting the digestive system. Here are detailed explanations of the process, potential risks, recovery time, and potential complications associated with this procedure:

Process of Roux-en-Y Gastric Bypass (RYGB):

Preparation:

• Before surgery, patients undergo thorough evaluations, including medical assessments, nutritional counseling, and psychological evaluations.

• Patients are usually advised to follow a specific diet and lifestyle changes to reduce liver size, making the surgery safer.

Surgery:

• General anesthesia is administered to the patient.

• The surgeon makes several small incisions in the abdomen (laparoscopic approach) or a large incision (open surgery) to access the stomach and intestines.

• The surgeon staples the upper part of the stomach to create a small pouch, typically holding about one ounce of food.

• Next, the small intestine is divided, and the bottom end is connected to the small stomach pouch, forming the "Roux limb."

• The upper part of the divided small intestine is reattached further down the small intestine, forming the "Y limb," allowing digestive juices to mix with food further along the digestive tract.

• These rerouting bypasses a portion of the stomach and small intestine, reducing the amount of food the body can absorb and limiting caloric intake.

Risks and Potential Complications:

• Surgical Risks: Like any surgery, Roux-en-Y Gastric Bypass poses risks such as infection, bleeding, blood clots, or adverse reactions to anesthesia.

• Leakage or Fistula: A possible complication involves leaks at the surgical connections between the stomach and intestines, leading to leakage of stomach contents into the abdominal cavity.

• Nutritional Deficiencies: Patients may experience deficiencies in nutrients such as iron, vitamin B12, calcium, and others due to reduced absorption.

• Dumping Syndrome: Some patients may develop dumping syndrome, experiencing nausea, vomiting, weakness, or diarrhea after eating high-sugar or high-fat foods.

• Gallstones: Rapid weight loss after surgery can increase the risk of gallstone formation.

Recovery Time:

• Hospital Stay: Most patients stay in the hospital for 2 to 3 days after surgery.

• Return to Normal Activities: Recovery varies, but patients may resume light activities within a few weeks.

• Diet Progression: Patients start with a liquid diet, gradually transitioning to pureed foods, soft foods, and eventually solid foods over several weeks.

Long-Term Considerations:

• Lifestyle Changes: Patients need to adhere to strict dietary guidelines and commit to lifelong changes in eating habits and exercise routines.

• Regular Follow-ups: Follow-up appointments with healthcare providers are crucial to monitor weight loss, nutritional status, and address any concerns or complications.

Roux-en-Y Gastric Bypass is an effective weight-loss surgery, but it involves significant lifestyle changes and potential risks. Patients considering this procedure should have a thorough understanding of the process, potential complications, and commit to post-operative care and lifestyle modifications for successful outcomes. Consulting with healthcare professionals is essential for personalized guidance and support throughout the surgical process and recovery.

Mini-Gastric Bypass (MGB) is a type of weight-loss surgery that involves creating a smaller stomach pouch and rerouting the digestive tract. Here's an overview of the process, potential risks, recovery time, and potential complications associated with Mini-Gastric Bypass:

Process of Mini-Gastric Bypass (MGB):

Preparation:

• Patients undergo comprehensive medical evaluations, including assessments of overall health and nutritional status.

• Pre-surgery dietary changes and lifestyle modifications may be recommended to prepare for the procedure.

Surgery:

• General anesthesia is administered to the patient.

• The surgeon makes small incisions in the abdomen (usually employing a laparoscopic approach) to access the stomach and intestines.

• A longer and narrower stomach pouch is created, typically along the lesser curvature of the stomach, reducing its capacity.

• The small intestine is divided and attached to the newly created stomach pouch, allowing food to bypass a portion of the small intestine.

• The procedure reroutes the digestive tract, limiting the amount of food that can be consumed and altering nutrient absorption.

• Surgical Risks: As with any surgery, risks include infection, bleeding, blood clots, and adverse reactions to anesthesia.

• Leakage or Fistula: There is a risk of leakage or fistula at the surgical connections between the stomach and intestines, leading to the leakage of stomach contents.

• Nutritional Deficiencies: Reduced absorption may lead to deficiencies in essential nutrients such as vitamins and minerals.

• Dumping Syndrome: Some patients may experience symptoms like nausea, vomiting, weakness, and diarrhea after consuming high-sugar or high-fat foods.

• Gallstones: Rapid weight loss following surgery may increase the risk of gallstone formation.

Recovery Time:

• Hospital Stay: Patients typically stay in the hospital for 1 to 2 days after Mini-Gastric Bypass surgery.

• Return to Normal Activities: Recovery time varies, but most individuals can resume light activities within a few weeks.

• Diet Progression: Patients start with a liquid diet, then transition to pureed foods, soft foods, and finally solid foods over several weeks.

Long-Term Considerations:

• Lifestyle Changes: Patients need to adhere to dietary guidelines and commit to lifelong changes in eating habits and regular exercise routines.

• Follow-up Care: Regular follow-up appointments with healthcare providers are essential to monitor weight loss progress, nutritional status, and address any post-operative concerns or complications.

Mini-Gastric Bypass is a weight-loss surgery offering potential benefits, but it requires careful consideration of the associated risks and commitment to post-operative care and lifestyle modifications. Individuals considering this procedure should consult healthcare professionals for personalized guidance and support throughout the surgical process and recovery. As with any surgical intervention, understanding the process and potential complications is crucial in making informed decisions about this procedure.

THE PROCESS, RISKS, RECOVERY TIME, AND POTENTIAL COMPLICATIONS OF BILIOPANCREATIC DIVERSION WITH DUODENAL SWITCH.

Biliopancreatic Diversion with Duodenal Switch (BPD-DS) is a complex weight-loss surgery involving two steps: a sleeve gastrectomy followed by rerouting of the small intestine to achieve weight loss. Here's a detailed explanation of the process, potential risks, recovery time, and potential complications associated with BPD-DS:

Process of Biliopancreatic Diversion with Duodenal Switch (BPD-DS):

Preparation:

• Patients undergo thorough evaluations, including medical assessments, nutritional counseling, and psychological evaluations.

• Pre-surgery dietary changes and lifestyle modifications may be recommended to optimize health before the procedure.

First Step: Sleeve Gastrectomy:

• A portion (about 70-80%) of the stomach is removed, creating a smaller, banana-shaped stomach pouch, restricting the amount of food that can be consumed.

Second Step: Intestinal Rerouting:

• The surgeon divides the small intestine and connects the end of the small intestine directly to the duodenum (the first part of the small intestine) near the stomach, bypassing a significant portion of the small intestine.

• This rerouting limits the path food travels, reducing calorie and nutrient absorption.

Risks and Potential Complications:

• Surgical Risks: Common risks associated with any surgery, including infection, bleeding, blood clots, or adverse reactions to anesthesia.

• Leakage or Fistula: There's a risk of leaks at the surgical connections or the staple line, leading to the leakage of stomach contents into the abdominal cavity.

• Nutritional Deficiencies: Reduced absorption can cause deficiencies in essential nutrients, including vitamins (such as A, D, E, K) and minerals (such as iron and calcium).

• Dumping Syndrome: Some patients may experience symptoms like nausea, vomiting, weakness, and diarrhea after eating certain foods high in sugar or fat.

• Gallstones: Rapid weight loss may increase the risk of developing gallstones.

Recovery Time:

• Hospital Stay: Patients typically stay in the hospital for 2 to 4 days after BPD-DS surgery.

• Return to Normal Activities: Recovery varies, but most individuals can resume light activities within a few weeks.

• Diet Progression: Patients start with a liquid diet, progress to pureed foods, soft foods, and eventually solid foods over several weeks to months.

Long-Term Considerations:

• Lifestyle Changes: Patients need to adhere strictly to dietary guidelines, take prescribed supplements, and commit to lifelong changes in eating habits and regular exercise routines.

• Follow-up Care: Regular follow-up appointments with healthcare providers are crucial to monitor weight loss, nutritional status, and address any post-operative complications or deficiencies.

Biliopancreatic Diversion with Duodenal Switch is a highly effective weight-loss surgery but is complex and carries potential risks and long-term considerations. Patients considering this procedure should have a comprehensive understanding of the process, potential complications, and commit to post-operative care and lifestyle modifications. Consulting with healthcare professionals is essential for personalized guidance and support throughout the surgical process and recovery.

Loop gastric bypass, also known as Single-Anastomosis Duodenal-Ileal Bypass with Sleeve Gastrectomy (SADI-S), is a type of weight-loss surgery that combines elements of sleeve gastrectomy and gastric bypass to aid in weight reduction. Here's an in-depth explanation of the process, potential risks, recovery time, and potential complications associated with loop gastric bypass:

Process of Loop Gastric Bypass (SADI-S):

Preparation:

• Patients undergo comprehensive evaluations, including medical assessments, nutritional counseling, and psychological evaluations.

• Pre-surgery dietary changes and lifestyle modifications may be recommended to optimize health before the procedure.

Surgery:

• General anesthesia is administered to the patient.

• The surgeon performs a sleeve gastrectomy, removing a portion (about 70-80%) of the stomach to create a smaller stomach pouch.

• Next, the small intestine is divided, and one end is connected to the duodenum (first part of the small intestine) and the other end is connected to the ileum (further down the small intestine).

• This rerouting allows food to bypass a significant portion of the small intestine, limiting calorie and nutrient absorption.

Risks and Potential Complications:

• Surgical Risks: Common risks associated with any surgery, such as infection, bleeding, blood clots, or adverse reactions to anesthesia.

• Leakage or Fistula: There's a risk of leaks at the surgical connections or the staple line, leading to the leakage of stomach contents.

• Nutritional Deficiencies: Reduced absorption can cause deficiencies in essential nutrients, including vitamins (such as A, D, E, K) and minerals (such as iron and calcium).

• Dumping Syndrome: Some patients may experience symptoms like nausea, vomiting, weakness, and diarrhea after eating certain foods high in sugar or fat.

• Gallstones: Rapid weight loss may increase the risk of developing gallstones.

Recovery Time:

• Hospital Stay: Patients typically stay in the hospital for 2 to 3 days after loop gastric bypass surgery.

• Return to Normal Activities: Recovery varies, but most individuals can resume light activities within a few weeks.

• Diet Progression: Patients start with a liquid diet, progress to pureed foods, soft foods, and eventually solid foods over several weeks to months.

• Lifestyle Changes: Patients need to adhere strictly to dietary guidelines, take prescribed supplements, and commit to lifelong changes in eating habits and regular exercise routines.

• Follow-up Care: Regular follow-up appointments with healthcare providers are crucial to monitor weight loss, nutritional status, and address any post-operative complications or deficiencies.

Loop gastric bypass (SADI-S) is a relatively new and effective weight-loss surgery, but like any surgical procedure, it involves potential risks and long-term considerations. Patients considering this procedure should have a thorough understanding of the process, potential complications, and commit to post-operative care and lifestyle modifications. Consulting with healthcare professionals is essential for personalized guidance and support throughout the surgical process and recovery.

THE STEPS PATIENTS SHOULD TAKE BEFORE GASTRIC BYPASS SURGERY

Before undergoing gastric bypass surgery, patients should follow specific steps and guidelines to ensure their safety, readiness for the procedure, and optimize the chances of a successful outcome. Here are detailed steps patients should take before gastric bypass surgery:

1. Consultation and Evaluation:

• Medical Evaluation: Undergo comprehensive medical assessments, including physical examinations, blood tests, imaging studies, and cardiac evaluations, to assess overall health and identify any underlying medical conditions.

• Nutritional Assessment: Consult with a registered dietitian or nutritionist to evaluate current dietary habits, discuss nutritional deficiencies, and plan a pre-operative diet to optimize nutrition and reduce liver size.

• Psychological Evaluation: Attend a psychological evaluation to assess mental health, evaluate readiness for surgery, and discuss expectations, coping mechanisms, and post-operative lifestyle changes.

2. Lifestyle Modifications:

• Dietary Changes: Follow a prescribed pre-operative diet that may include reducing calorie intake, increasing protein intake, and avoiding high-calorie or high-fat foods. This diet often aims to shrink the liver and facilitate easier surgery.

• Exercise Routine: Engage in regular physical activity as advised by healthcare providers to improve fitness levels and optimize overall health before surgery.

• Smoking and Alcohol Cessation: Quit smoking and limit alcohol intake as recommended by healthcare professionals. Smoking cessation helps improve healing and reduces the risk of complications.

3. Education and Preparation:

• Attend Pre-operative Education Sessions: Participate in educational sessions or seminars provided by the surgical team to understand the procedure, post-operative expectations, dietary changes, and potential risks and complications.

• Medication Review: Review all current medications with the healthcare team to determine which medications need to be adjusted, stopped, or continued before surgery.

• Pre-operative Testing: Complete all necessary pre-operative tests and screenings, such as blood tests, imaging studies, and cardiac evaluations, as recommended by healthcare providers.

4. Psychological Readiness:

• Understanding Expectations: Have a clear understanding of the expected outcomes, lifestyle changes, and commitment required post-surgery for successful weight loss and improved health.

• Support System: Establish a strong support system of family members, friends, or support groups to provide emotional support and assistance during the pre-operative and post-operative periods.

5. Compliance with Guidelines:

• Follow Healthcare Provider Instructions: Adhere strictly to pre-operative instructions provided by the healthcare team regarding diet, medications, and lifestyle modifications.

• Maintain Communication: Maintain open communication with the healthcare team, addressing any concerns or questions before the surgery.

By following these steps and guidelines before gastric bypass surgery, patients can prepare themselves physically, mentally, and emotionally for the procedure, reducing potential risks and optimizing the likelihood of a successful surgery and recovery. It's crucial to work closely with healthcare professionals and adhere to their recommendations throughout the pre-operative process.

STAGES OF RECOVERY OF GASTRIC BYPASS SURGERY

The recovery process following gastric bypass surgery involves several stages as the body heals and adjusts to the surgical changes. Here's an overview of the typical stages of recovery:

Immediate Post-Surgery (Hospital Stay):

• Hospitalization: Patients usually spend 1-3 days in the hospital after surgery, depending on their recovery progress and the specific surgical approach.

• Monitoring: Medical staff monitor vital signs, manage pain, and ensure patients can tolerate liquids before discharge.

• Initial Diet: Introduction to clear liquids, gradually progressing to full liquids before transitioning to pureed or soft foods.

First Few Weeks at Home:

• Transitioning Diet: Patients follow a gradual diet progression, advancing from pureed foods to soft solids over several weeks.

• Pain Management: Managing incision site pain and discomfort with prescribed medications and following post-operative care instructions.

• Limited Physical Activity: Initially restricted from strenuous activities and heavy lifting, gradually increasing movement and walking as tolerated.

Weeks 4-6:

• Improved Dietary Intake: Transitioning to a wider variety of foods while adhering to portion control and dietary guidelines.

• Follow-up Appointments: Scheduled follow-up visits with the surgeon or healthcare team to monitor progress, address concerns, and assess nutritional status.

• Increasing Activity Levels: Encouraged to engage in light exercises or activities based on the healthcare provider's recommendations.

Months 2-6:

• Establishing Routine: Settling into a regular eating pattern, focusing on nutrient-dense foods and portion control.

• Gradual Exercise Increase: Gradually incorporating more structured exercise routines, including aerobic and strength training, based on recovery progress.

• Psychological Adjustment: Working through emotional and psychological aspects of the weight loss journey, potentially seeking counseling or support groups.

Beyond 6 Months:

• Long-Term Lifestyle Changes: Embracing a sustainable, healthy lifestyle with continued focus on diet, exercise, and psychological well-being.

• **Regular Follow-ups:** Continuing regular check-ups with healthcare providers for monitoring weight loss, nutritional status, and overall health.

• **Support Network:** Building a support network, staying engaged in follow-up care, and seeking professional guidance as needed for long-term success.

Recovery from gastric bypass surgery is a gradual process, and the timeline can vary for each individual. It's essential to follow healthcare provider recommendations, adhere to dietary guidelines, engage in physical activity, and seek support to ensure a smooth recovery and successful long-term outcomes.

GUIDANCE ON DIET PROGRESSION POST-SURGERY RECOVERY

The diet progression following gastric bypass surgery involves gradual stages to allow the stomach to heal, adapt to its new size, and reintroduce foods as the patient's tolerance improves. Please note that the diet progression may vary based on the surgeon's recommendations and individual patient needs. Here's a general guideline for diet progression post-surgery recovery:

Phase 1: Clear Liquid Diet (Days 1-7):

Objective: Prevent dehydration and provide hydration.

Allowed Foods:

• Clear liquids such as water, broth, sugar-free gelatin, and sugar-free popsicles.

• Protein supplements (as recommended by the healthcare provider).

Guidelines:

• Sip fluids slowly throughout the day to stay hydrated.

• Avoid carbonated beverages and caffeine.

• Aim to consume small amounts frequently to prevent discomfort.

Phase 2: Full Liquid Diet (Days 8-14):

Objective: Gradually introduce more nutritional variety and aid in healing.

Allowed Foods:

• Clear liquids plus additional full liquids like low-fat yogurt, milk, protein shakes, and cream soups (strained without chunks).

Guidelines:

• Continue sipping liquids slowly.

• Focus on protein-rich liquids to aid in healing and muscle preservation.

• Avoid foods with added sugars or high-fat content.

Phase 3: Pureed or Blended Diet (Weeks 2-4):

Objective: Introduce pureed or blended foods to transition toward a more varied diet.

Allowed Foods:

• Pureed or blended foods like cooked vegetables, soft fruits, lean ground meats, cottage cheese, and soft cereals.

Guidelines:

• Use a blender or food processor to create smooth textures without lumps.

• Consume small portions slowly and chew thoroughly.

• Avoid fibrous foods, tough meats, and foods that could cause discomfort or blockages.

Phase 4: Soft Solid Foods (Weeks 4 and Beyond):

Objective: Gradually introduce soft solid foods while continuing to avoid foods that may cause discomfort or blockages.

Allowed Foods:

• Soft, well-cooked foods like fish, tender chicken, tofu, cooked vegetables, ripe fruits, and whole grains.

Guidelines:

• Chew food thoroughly and eat slowly to aid digestion and prevent discomfort.

• Focus on protein-rich foods to promote healing and muscle maintenance.

• Continue avoiding high-sugar, high-fat, or carbonated foods and drinks.

Additional Tips:

• Hydration: Continue to prioritize hydration by sipping water throughout the day.

• Portion Control: Focus on smaller, frequent meals to prevent overeating and discomfort.

• Supplements: Follow recommendations for prescribed vitamins and mineral supplements to prevent deficiencies.

• Listen to Your Body: Pay attention to signs of fullness or discomfort and adjust your eating habits accordingly.

Always consult with the healthcare provider or a registered dietitian for personalized dietary recommendations and guidelines tailored to your specific needs and recovery progress following gastric bypass surgery.

PHYSICAL ACTIVITY POST-SURGERY RECOVERY

Physical activity post-gastric bypass surgery is a crucial component of the recovery process and plays a significant role in enhancing overall health, aiding in weight loss, and promoting long-term success. However, it's essential to start gradually and follow specific guidelines to ensure safety and prevent complications. Here's guidance on physical activity during the recovery period after gastric bypass surgery:

1. Follow Healthcare Provider's Recommendations:

• Consultation: Seek guidance from the healthcare team before initiating any exercise routine.

• Individualized Plan: Discuss an individualized exercise plan based on your health condition, fitness level, and recovery progress.

2. Early Post-Surgery Phase (Days to Weeks):

• Light Activity: Begin with short, gentle walks around the house or short walks outdoors, depending on your comfort level.

• Gradual Progression: Increase activity gradually, starting with 5-10 minute sessions a few times a day and slowly increasing duration as tolerated.

• Avoid Strain: Avoid heavy lifting, strenuous activities, or activities that strain the abdominal area.

3. Intermediate Phase (Weeks to Months):

• Low-Impact Exercises: Engage in low-impact activities such as walking, swimming, stationary cycling, or using an elliptical machine.

• Increase Duration: Gradually extend exercise sessions to 20-30 minutes, aiming for at least 150 minutes of moderate-intensity exercise per week.

• Strength Training: Incorporate light strength training with resistance bands or light weights to maintain muscle mass.

4. Long-Term Maintenance (Months and Beyond):

• Variety: Include a variety of exercises to maintain interest and engage different muscle groups.

• Increase Intensity: Gradually increase the intensity of workouts, incorporating moderate to vigorous exercises based on your tolerance.

• Consistency: Aim for regular physical activity sessions, striving for at least 30 minutes of exercise most days of the week.

Additional Tips:

• Listen to Your Body: Pay attention to how your body responds to exercise and avoid pushing yourself too hard.

• Stay Hydrated: Drink plenty of water before, during, and after exercising to prevent dehydration.

• Warm-up and Cool Down: Always start with a warm-up and end with a cool-down to prepare your body for exercise and reduce the risk of injury.

• Professional Guidance: Consider working with a certified fitness trainer or physical therapist to develop a safe and effective exercise program tailored to your needs.

Caution:

• Avoid High-Impact Activities: Steer clear of high-impact exercises, especially in the early recovery phase, to prevent strain or injury to the surgical site.

• Report Discomfort: If you experience severe pain, unusual symptoms, or discomfort during or after exercise, stop immediately and consult your healthcare provider.

Always remember that the recovery process after gastric bypass surgery varies for each individual. Prioritize safety, gradual progression, and regular communication with healthcare providers to ensure a safe and effective exercise routine during your recovery period and beyond.

CHAPTER TWO

PAIN MANAGEMENT POST-SURGERY RECOVERY

Pain management is an essential aspect of post-surgery recovery after gastric bypass surgery. Adequate pain control promotes comfort, facilitates mobility, and supports a smoother recovery process. Here's guidance on pain management during the post-surgery recovery period:

1. Follow Healthcare Provider's Instructions:

• Medications: Take prescribed pain medications as directed by your healthcare provider. Follow the recommended dosage and schedule to manage pain effectively.

• Ask Questions: Seek clarification on how to take pain medications, potential side effects, and when to contact the healthcare provider regarding concerns.

2. Use Ice Packs or Heat Therapy:

• Ice Packs: Applying ice packs (wrapped in a cloth) to the surgical site can help reduce swelling and alleviate discomfort.

• Heat Therapy: Heat packs or warm compresses may also provide relief for muscle soreness or discomfort. Ensure the incision area is healed before using heat therapy.

3. Positioning and Rest:

• Proper Rest: Ensure adequate rest and sleep to support the healing process. Find a comfortable sleeping position that minimizes pressure on the surgical area.

• Pillow Support: Use pillows to support your body while lying down, sitting, or moving to alleviate discomfort.

4. Gentle Movement and Mobility:

• Early Movement: Engage in gentle movements and short walks as advised by the healthcare provider. Gradually increase activity levels as tolerated.

• Avoid Strain: Avoid heavy lifting or strenuous activities that might strain the abdominal area or surgical incisions.

5. Relaxation Techniques:

• Breathing Exercises: Practice deep breathing exercises or relaxation techniques to reduce stress, relax muscles, and manage discomfort.

• Mindfulness: Mindfulness meditation or guided imagery may help distract from pain and promote relaxation.

6. Nutrition and Hydration:

• Balanced Diet: Follow the recommended diet plan provided by the healthcare team, as proper nutrition supports healing and recovery.

• Hydration: Drink plenty of fluids (except carbonated beverages) to stay hydrated and support the healing process.

7. Communicate with Healthcare Providers:

• Report Pain Levels: Inform your healthcare provider about your pain levels, any changes in symptoms, or concerns about pain management.

• Ask for Help: If pain persists or worsens, seek medical attention promptly. Do not hesitate to ask for assistance or guidance from healthcare professionals.

8. Patience and Expectations:

• Recovery Time: Understand that pain and discomfort are common after surgery but should gradually improve over time. Be patient with the recovery process.

• Set Realistic Expectations: Everyone's pain experience and recovery timeline are different. Focus on gradual progress rather than expecting immediate relief.

Caution:

• Avoid Self-Medication: Do not take additional medications or alter prescribed dosages without consulting your healthcare provider.

• Watch for Warning Signs: Monitor for signs of infection (increased redness, warmth, swelling, or discharge at the incision site) and report to your doctor immediately if observed.

Always follow the guidance provided by your healthcare team and communicate openly about your pain levels and recovery progress. Effective pain management strategies can help alleviate discomfort and support a smoother recovery following gastric bypass surgery.

PSYCHOLOGICAL ADJUSTMENTS DURING THE RECOVERY PHASE

Psychological adjustments during the recovery phase after gastric bypass surgery are as crucial as physical recovery. The procedure often involves significant lifestyle changes and emotional adjustments. Here's guidance to help navigate the psychological aspects of recovery:

1. Embrace Realistic Expectations:

• Understanding Change: Recognize that the recovery period involves both physical and emotional adjustments. Understand that changes in lifestyle and body image take time.

2. Accept Emotional Changes:

• Mood Swings: Be prepared for potential mood swings or emotional fluctuations post-surgery due to hormonal changes, stress, or adjustments to dietary habits.

• Seek Support: Talk openly about your emotions with trusted friends, family, or a support group. Sharing your feelings can help relieve emotional stress.

3. Patience with Weight Loss:

• Gradual Progress: Understand that weight loss after surgery is gradual and varies among individuals. Avoid comparing your progress to others.

• Focus on Health: Shift the focus from rapid weight loss to overall health improvements and adopting a sustainable lifestyle.

4. Body Image Concerns:

• Adjusting Body Image: Be patient with changes in body image as weight loss progresses. Give yourself time to adapt to your changing appearance.

• Self-Acceptance: Focus on self-acceptance and celebrate non-scale victories, such as increased energy levels or improved health markers.

5. Behavioral Changes:

• Eating Habits: Adjusting to new eating habits can be challenging. Work with a dietitian or counselor to navigate changes and develop a healthy relationship with food.

• Mindful Eating: Practice mindful eating, focusing on hunger cues and eating for nourishment rather than emotional reasons.

6. Set Realistic Goals:

• Achievable Goals: Set achievable short-term and long-term goals for lifestyle changes, physical activity, and overall well-being.

• Celebrate Progress: Acknowledge and celebrate milestones achieved in your recovery journey, no matter how small.

7. Seek Professional Support:

• Therapy or Counseling: Consider therapy or counseling sessions with a mental health professional specializing in bariatric surgery or weight management.

• Support Groups: Join support groups or attend meetings where you can connect with others who have undergone similar experiences.

8. Self-Care and Stress Management:

• Prioritize Self-Care: Engage in activities that promote relaxation, such as meditation, deep breathing exercises, yoga, or hobbies you enjoy.

• Stress Reduction: Manage stress through healthy coping mechanisms like journaling, walking, or engaging in activities that bring joy.

9. Be Patient and Kind to Yourself:

• Recovery Takes Time: Understand that recovery, both physically and emotionally, is a process that takes time. Be patient and kind to yourself throughout the journey.

• Seek Help When Needed: If feelings of anxiety, depression, or stress persist, seek professional help without hesitation.

Gastric bypass surgery involves significant lifestyle changes and emotional adjustments. It's crucial to acknowledge and address these psychological aspects to achieve successful long-term outcomes. Surround yourself with supportive individuals, seek professional guidance when needed, and prioritize self-care during your recovery journey.

LONG-TERM DIETARY MODIFICATIONS NECESSARY FOR MAINTAINING WEIGHT LOSS AND OVERALL HEALTH AFTER GASTRIC BYPASS SURGERY

Long-term dietary modifications are crucial after gastric bypass surgery to maintain weight loss, support overall health, and prevent nutritional deficiencies. Here's a detailed discussion on the dietary changes required for long-term success:

1. Emphasis on Nutrient-Dense Foods:

• Lean Proteins: Prioritize lean protein sources like poultry, fish, tofu, legumes, and low-fat dairy to support muscle maintenance and satiety.

• Vegetables and Fruits: Consume a variety of colorful vegetables and fruits for essential vitamins, minerals, fiber, and antioxidants.

• Whole Grains: Incorporate whole grains like quinoa, brown rice, oats, and whole wheat for sustained energy and fiber.

2. Portion Control and Meal Structure:

• Small, Frequent Meals: Continue eating small, balanced meals throughout the day to prevent overeating and promote steady energy levels.

• Avoid Grazing: Avoid continuous snacking or grazing between meals to maintain portion control.

• Chew Thoroughly: Chew food slowly and thoroughly to aid digestion and prevent discomfort.

3. Hydration and Fluid Intake:

• Water Consumption: Stay well-hydrated by drinking water throughout the day. Avoid high-calorie beverages, sugary drinks, and excessive caffeine.

• Avoid Drinking with Meals: Refrain from drinking fluids with meals to prevent discomfort and ensure adequate nutrient absorption.

4. Nutritional Supplements:

• Follow Prescribed Supplements: Take prescribed vitamins and mineral supplements regularly to prevent deficiencies due to reduced absorption.

• Monitoring Nutrient Levels: Periodically monitor nutrient levels through blood tests as advised by healthcare professionals.

5. Mindful Eating and Behavior Changes:

• Mindful Eating Practices: Practice mindful eating, focusing on hunger cues and recognizing fullness to prevent overeating.

• Avoid Emotional Eating: Develop strategies to manage emotions without resorting to food, seeking alternative coping mechanisms.

6. Avoid Trigger Foods and Unhealthy Choices:

• Identify Trigger Foods: Recognize and avoid high-calorie, high-sugar, or high-fat trigger foods that may lead to overeating or discomfort.

• Limit Processed Foods: Reduce intake of processed and refined foods, aiming for whole, unprocessed options for better nutrition.

7. Regular Monitoring and Professional Guidance:

• Regular Follow-ups: Attend regular follow-up appointments with healthcare providers for nutritional assessments, weight monitoring, and guidance.

• Registered Dietitian Support: Consult with a registered dietitian specializing in bariatric nutrition for personalized guidance and meal planning.

8. Lifestyle Integration:

• Healthy Cooking Methods: Opt for healthier cooking methods like grilling, baking, steaming, or sautéing instead of frying.

• Balanced Eating Habits: Focus on balanced meals containing adequate protein, healthy fats, and fiber-rich carbohydrates for sustained energy.

• Cultivate Healthy Habits: Create an environment that supports healthy eating, mindful behaviors, and an active lifestyle.

Long-term success after gastric bypass surgery relies heavily on adopting and maintaining healthy eating habits, portion control, and mindful choices. Consistency, regular monitoring, and seeking professional guidance when needed are key components for sustained weight loss and overall health.

LONG-TERM EXERCISE ROUTINES NECESSARY FOR MAINTAINING WEIGHT LOSS AND OVERALL HEALTH AFTER GASTRIC BYPASS SURGERY

Incorporating long-term exercise routines after gastric bypass surgery is vital for maintaining weight loss, improving overall health, and sustaining a healthy lifestyle. Here's a detailed discussion on the exercise strategies necessary for long-term success:

1. Aerobic/Cardiovascular Exercise:

• Moderate Intensity: Aim for at least 150 minutes of moderate-intensity aerobic exercise per week, such as brisk walking, cycling, or swimming.

• Variety: Incorporate various activities like dancing, jogging, or using cardio machines to prevent boredom and engage different muscle groups.

• Interval Training: Implement interval training by alternating between periods of high intensity and low intensity to enhance calorie burning and cardiovascular fitness.

2. Strength Training/Resistance Exercises:

• Muscle Maintenance: Include strength training exercises 2-3 times a week to preserve and build muscle mass, which can decline during weight loss.

• Bodyweight Exercises: Incorporate bodyweight exercises (push-ups, squats, lunges) or use resistance bands, free weights, or weight machines for strength training.

• Focus on Major Muscle Groups: Target major muscle groups including chest, back, legs, shoulders, arms, and core.

3. Flexibility and Stretching:

• Stretching Routine: Perform stretching exercises regularly to improve flexibility and prevent muscle tightness or injury.

• Yoga or Pilates: Consider yoga or Pilates sessions to enhance flexibility, core strength, and relaxation.

4. Daily Physical Activity:

• Active Lifestyle: Incorporate physical activity into daily routines, such as taking the stairs, walking during breaks, or doing household chores.

• Pedometer or Activity Tracker: Use a pedometer or activity tracker to monitor daily steps and motivate yourself to increase physical activity levels gradually.

5. Outdoor Activities and Recreation:

• Nature Walks/Hiking: Explore outdoor activities like nature walks, hiking, or trail walking to enjoy fresh air and diverse terrain.

• Recreational Sports: Participate in recreational sports leagues or activities such as tennis, basketball, or group fitness classes for enjoyment and social interaction.

6. Consistency and Progression:

• Consistent Routine: Establish a regular exercise routine and aim for consistency in daily or weekly workouts.

• Gradual Progression: Gradually increase exercise intensity, duration, or types of workouts to challenge yourself and avoid plateaus.

7. Mindful Movement:

• Mind-Body Exercises: Engage in mind-body exercises like tai chi or qigong for relaxation, balance, and mind-body connection.

• Focus on Form: Pay attention to proper form and technique during exercises to prevent injury and maximize effectiveness.

8. Professional Guidance and Safety:

• Consultation with Experts: Seek guidance from fitness trainers, physical therapists, or healthcare professionals to design a safe and effective exercise program tailored to your needs.

• Listen to Your Body: Pay attention to your body's signals and limitations. If you experience pain or discomfort, modify exercises or consult a professional.

9. Lifestyle Integration:

• Consistent Activity: Make physical activity a regular part of your lifestyle, integrating it into your daily routine for long-term sustainability.

• Variety and Enjoyment: Choose activities you enjoy and vary your workouts to prevent monotony and sustain motivation.

Long-term success after gastric bypass surgery requires a commitment to regular exercise, including a mix of aerobic, strength, flexibility, and daily activities. Always prioritize safety, listen to your body, and seek professional guidance to develop a well-rounded and sustainable exercise routine that supports your weight loss and overall health goals.

COMMON ISSUES POST-SURGERY

Here are some common issues individuals may face post-gastric bypass surgery along with coping strategies and potential solutions:

Dumping Syndrome:

Issue: Rapid emptying of the stomach contents into the small intestine, causing nausea, weakness, sweating, and diarrhea after consuming certain foods high in sugar or fat.

Coping Strategies:

• Diet Modification: Avoid high-sugar and high-fat foods that trigger dumping syndrome.

• Eat Smaller, Frequent Meals: Opt for smaller meals throughout the day to prevent overloading the digestive system.

• Stay Hydrated: Sip water between meals to maintain hydration without affecting digestion.

Nutritional Deficiencies:

Issue: Reduced absorption of nutrients, leading to deficiencies in vitamins (like B12, D, iron) and minerals (like calcium).

Coping Strategies:

• Supplements: Take prescribed vitamin and mineral supplements regularly as advised by healthcare providers.

• Regular Monitoring: Periodic blood tests to monitor nutrient levels and adjust supplements accordingly.

Emotional Eating or Psychological Challenges:

Issue: Coping with emotional triggers or using food as a source of comfort, leading to overeating.

Coping Strategies:

• Therapy or Support Groups: Attend counseling or support groups to address emotional challenges and learn healthier coping mechanisms.

• Mindfulness Techniques: Practice mindfulness, meditation, or deep breathing exercises to manage stress and emotions without turning to food.

• Keep a Food Diary: Monitor and track food intake, emotional triggers, and feelings associated with eating to identify patterns and seek alternative coping strategies.

Plateaus in Weight Loss:

Issue: Periods where weight loss stalls despite adhering to diet and exercise routines.

Coping Strategies:

• Change Exercise Routine: Modify and diversify exercise routines to challenge the body differently.

• Review Diet Habits: Reassess portion sizes, food choices, and overall diet to ensure compliance with recommended guidelines.

• Consult Professionals: Seek guidance from healthcare providers or dietitians to evaluate and adjust the weight loss plan if necessary.

Body Image and Self-Esteem Issues:

Issue: Adjusting to changes in body appearance and dealing with self-esteem issues after significant weight loss.

Coping Strategies:

• Seek Support: Join support groups or counseling sessions to discuss body image concerns and receive guidance.

• Focus on Non-Scale Victories: Celebrate achievements beyond weight loss, such as increased energy, improved fitness, or better health markers.

Regaining Weight:

Issue: Some individuals may experience weight regain after initial successful weight loss.

Coping Strategies:

• Mindful Eating: Revisit mindful eating practices and focus on portion control and healthy food choices.

• Physical Activity: Increase or modify exercise routines to boost metabolism and aid weight maintenance.

• Professional Guidance: Consult healthcare professionals or a dietitian for personalized advice and support.

Social and Lifestyle Adjustments:

Issue: Navigating social situations or lifestyle changes concerning eating habits after surgery.

Coping Strategies:

• Communicate Openly: Communicate your dietary needs and limitations with friends and family to avoid uncomfortable situations.

• Plan Ahead: Plan meals and snacks in advance when attending events or social gatherings to ensure healthier choices are available.

For any specific concerns or complications post-surgery, it's essential to consult with healthcare professionals or specialists who can provide personalized guidance and solutions tailored to individual needs. Building a support network, staying informed, and implementing coping strategies are vital for effectively managing common issues post-gastric bypass surgery.

MEAL PLANS CATERING FOR THE FIRST FEW WEEKS AT HOME

During the first few weeks at home after gastric bypass surgery, the diet typically progresses from full liquids to pureed foods and soft solids. Here are sample meal plans catering to this initial phase of recovery:

Week 1-2: Full Liquids to Pureed Foods

Day 1-3: Full Liquids

• Breakfast: Protein-fortified low-sugar shake or smoothie (unsweetened almond milk or low-fat yogurt)

• Snack: Broth-based soups (strained to remove solids)

• Lunch: Blended vegetable or chicken soup (strained)

• Snack: Sugar-free gelatin or pudding

• Dinner: Creamy soups (strained)

Day 4-7: Transition to Pureed Foods

• Breakfast: Blended oatmeal or cream of wheat (cooked until very soft)

• Snack: Greek yogurt blended with fruit or unsweetened applesauce

• Lunch: Pureed chicken or fish with steamed vegetables (blended to a smooth consistency)

• Snack: Protein-fortified pudding or cottage cheese (blended)

• Dinner: Pureed bean or lentil soup

Week 3-4: Pureed Foods to Soft Solids

Day 8-14: Transitioning to Soft Solids

- Breakfast: Soft scrambled eggs or tofu with spinach

- Snack: Soft fruits like bananas or ripe avocado

- Lunch: Soft-textured fish or tofu with cooked vegetables

- Snack: Hummus with whole-grain crackers or soft cheese

- Dinner: Ground turkey or chicken with mashed sweet potatoes

Day 15-21: Soft Solids Introduction

- Breakfast: Poached eggs with whole-grain toast (cut into small pieces)

- Snack: Cottage cheese or Greek yogurt with fruit chunks

- Lunch: Baked or grilled chicken with steamed vegetables (cut into small pieces)

- Snack: Apple sauce or fruit compote

- Dinner: Soft-textured fish or tofu with quinoa or mashed cauliflower

General Tips:

- Portion Control: Continue with small, frequent meals to avoid overeating.

• Protein Intake: Prioritize lean proteins to aid healing and maintain muscle mass.

• Hydration: Sip water regularly between meals to maintain hydration levels.

• Avoid Straining Foods: Avoid tough or fibrous foods that may be difficult to digest.

Always adhere to the dietary guidelines provided by your healthcare team and progress through the diet stages at your own pace based on individual tolerance levels. Consult with a dietitian or healthcare professional for personalized meal plans adapted to your recovery needs.

MEAL PLANS CATERING FOR WEEKS 4-6 AT HOME

During weeks 4-6 after gastric bypass surgery, individuals typically progress to a wider variety of foods while still focusing on pureed and soft textures. Here's a sample meal plan catering to this stage of recovery:

Week 4-6: Advanced Pureed and Soft Solids

Day 1-3: Advanced Pureed Foods

Breakfast:

• Greek yogurt blended with soft fruits (like berries or banana)

• Protein-fortified oatmeal (blended for a smoother texture)

Snack:

• Cottage cheese or ricotta cheese with applesauce or mashed fruits

Lunch:

• Pureed chicken or turkey chili

• Blended vegetable soup with added protein (chicken or beans)

Snack:

• Protein-fortified pudding or smoothie

Dinner:

• Mashed cauliflower with pureed white fish or tofu

• Pureed roasted vegetables (squash, carrots, or sweet potato)

Day 4-7: Introduction to Soft Solids

Breakfast:

• Scrambled eggs with sautéed spinach and mushrooms

• Soft whole-grain toast (small bites or well-soaked)

Snack:

• Sliced ripe avocado or mashed avocado on crackers

Lunch:

- Grilled or baked soft-textured chicken with steamed vegetables (cut into small pieces)

- Quinoa or mashed sweet potatoes

Snack:

- Fruit compote or fruit salad

Dinner:

- Soft-textured fish fillet (baked or grilled) with mashed cauliflower

- Blanched green beans or peas (softened)

General Tips:

- Texture Modification: Continue to focus on soft, easily chewable, and easily digestible foods.

- Portion Management: Stick to smaller, frequent meals to prevent discomfort and aid digestion.

- Nutrient Variety: Incorporate a variety of nutrient-dense foods to support overall health.

- Hydration: Stay hydrated by sipping water between meals.

As always, follow the dietary guidance provided by your healthcare team and advance through the diet stages based on individual tolerance levels. Consult with a dietitian or healthcare professional for personalized meal plans that align with your recovery needs.

During months 2-6 post-gastric bypass surgery, individuals can gradually introduce a wider variety of foods while focusing on nutrient-dense options and smaller portion sizes. Here's a sample meal plan catering to this stage of recovery:

Month 2-3: Transition to Soft Solid Foods

Day 1-3: Advanced Soft Solids

Breakfast:

• Scrambled eggs or tofu with sautéed vegetables (bell peppers, onions)

• Soft whole-grain toast or oatmeal with added nuts or seeds

Snack:

• Greek yogurt parfait with mixed berries and a sprinkle of granola

Lunch:

• Grilled or baked chicken breast with quinoa or brown rice

• Steamed or roasted vegetables (broccoli, cauliflower, carrots)

Snack:

• Hummus with veggie sticks or whole-grain crackers

Dinner:

• Baked fish with a side of mashed sweet potatoes

• Leafy green salad with soft lettuce, tomatoes, and a light vinaigrette

Day 4-7: Introduction of Whole Foods

Breakfast:

• Overnight oats with Greek yogurt, chia seeds, and fruit

• Soft-cooked poached eggs with whole-grain toast

Snack:

• Apple slices with nut butter or cottage cheese

Lunch:

• Grilled lean beef or tofu with quinoa salad (chopped vegetables mixed with quinoa)

• Steamed green beans or snap peas

Snack:

• Smoothie with protein powder, spinach, banana, and almond milk

Dinner:

• Roasted chicken or tofu stir-fry with mixed vegetables and brown rice

Month 4-6: Diversification and Balanced Meals

Day 1-3: Diversification of Meals

Breakfast:

• Veggie omelet with a side of whole-grain toast

• Greek yogurt parfait with nuts and fresh fruit

Snack:

• Trail mix (nuts, seeds, dried fruits)

Lunch:

• Grilled salmon or tofu with quinoa salad and roasted vegetables

• Mixed greens salad with assorted veggies, beans, and a light dressing

Snack:

• Protein-rich smoothie with mixed berries and spinach

Dinner:

• Turkey or black bean burgers with lettuce wraps or whole-grain buns

• Steamed or grilled vegetables with a side of couscous or bulgur

General Tips:

• Nutrient Density: Prioritize nutrient-dense foods and include a variety of lean proteins, whole grains, fruits, vegetables, and healthy fats.

• Portion Awareness: Continue practicing portion control and listening to hunger cues.

• Hydration: Maintain adequate hydration throughout the day.

• Slow Introductions: Introduce new foods gradually and observe how your body responds to them.

Adhere to dietary guidelines provided by your healthcare team, continue monitoring your progress, and seek guidance from a dietitian or healthcare professional for personalized meal plans adapted to your recovery needs and individual tolerances.

MEAL PLANS CATERING TO BEYOND 6 MONTHS POST-SURGERY

Beyond 6 months post-gastric bypass surgery, individuals can incorporate a wide range of nutrient-dense foods, maintaining smaller portion sizes and balanced meals. Here's a sample meal plan catering to this stage of recovery:

Day 1-3: Nutrient-Dense Meal Variety

Breakfast:

• Whole-grain toast with avocado, scrambled eggs, and a side of berries

• Greek yogurt parfait with nuts, seeds, and mixed fruit

Snack:

• Protein smoothie with spinach, protein powder, banana, and almond milk

Lunch:

• Grilled chicken or tofu salad with mixed greens, assorted veggies, and vinaigrette

• Quinoa or brown rice with grilled vegetables and lean protein

Snack:

• Cottage cheese with fresh fruit or whole-grain crackers

Dinner:

• Baked or grilled fish with a side of roasted sweet potatoes and steamed broccoli

• Stir-fried tofu or lean beef with colorful vegetables and whole-grain noodles

Breakfast:

• Smoothie bowl with blended fruit, yogurt, nuts, and seeds

• Veggie and cheese omelet with whole-grain toast

Snack:

• Apple slices with almond butter or a small handful of mixed nuts

Lunch:

• Quinoa and black bean salad with diced tomatoes, cucumbers, and lime vinaigrette

• Grilled shrimp or tempeh with a side of quinoa and steamed vegetables

Snack:

• Greek yogurt with granola and fresh berries

Dinner:

• Lean turkey or veggie meatballs with marinara sauce served over zucchini noodles

• Grilled chicken or portobello mushrooms with a side of roasted vegetables and a small portion of couscous

General Tips:

• Variety and Balance: Incorporate a variety of whole foods, lean proteins, healthy fats, fruits, vegetables, and whole grains.

• Portion Control: Continue practicing portion control to prevent overeating and aid digestion.

• Hydration: Ensure adequate hydration by drinking water throughout the day.

• Mindful Eating: Practice mindful eating by focusing on hunger cues and satiety signals.

Remember to follow the dietary guidance provided by your healthcare team, listen to your body's cues, and adapt your meal plan to meet your individual nutritional needs and preferences. Consulting with a dietitian or healthcare professional can help in creating personalized meal plans suitable for your continued recovery and long-term health.

THE DIETARY NEEDS POST-GASTRIC BYPASS SURGERY

Post-gastric bypass surgery, dietary needs change significantly due to the altered anatomy and reduced stomach capacity. Here are the key dietary needs to consider after gastric bypass surgery:

1. Protein Intake:

• Importance: Vital for tissue repair, healing, and preserving muscle mass after surgery.

• Recommendation: Consume lean protein sources such as poultry, fish, tofu, eggs, and legumes at each meal to meet daily protein needs.

2. Adequate Hydration:

• Importance: Maintain hydration to prevent dehydration and aid digestion.

• Recommendation: Sip water throughout the day, avoiding drinking with meals to prevent discomfort and ensure adequate hydration.

3. Vitamin and Mineral Supplements:

• Importance: Reduced absorption of nutrients post-surgery can lead to deficiencies.

• Recommendation: Follow prescribed supplements, including vitamins (B12, D, A, K) and minerals (iron, calcium) to prevent deficiencies.

4. Balanced Nutrition:

• Importance: Ensure a well-balanced diet to meet nutritional needs.

• Recommendation: Include a variety of fruits, vegetables, whole grains, and healthy fats to provide essential vitamins, minerals, and fiber.

5. Portion Control:

• Importance: Reduced stomach capacity requires smaller, more frequent meals.

• Recommendation: Consume small portions, chew food thoroughly, and avoid overeating to prevent discomfort and aid digestion.

6. Avoidance of Certain Foods:

• Importance: Some foods may cause discomfort or complications post-surgery.

• Recommendation: Avoid high-sugar, high-fat, carbonated, or fibrous foods that can cause dumping syndrome, digestive issues, or discomfort.

7. Gradual Diet Progression:

• Importance: Gradually reintroduce foods to allow the stomach to adapt.

• Recommendation: Follow the prescribed diet progression, starting from clear liquids, progressing to pureed foods, soft solids, and then gradually introducing regular textures.

8. Mindful Eating and Slow Eating Habits:

• Importance: Eating slowly aids digestion and prevents discomfort.

• Recommendation: Chew food thoroughly, eat mindfully, and stop eating when feeling comfortably full.

9. Regular Follow-up and Monitoring:

• Importance: Monitor weight, nutritional status, and overall health.

• Recommendation: Attend regular follow-up appointments with healthcare providers for nutritional assessments and adjustments as needed.

Following these dietary guidelines post-gastric bypass surgery is essential for optimal recovery, ensuring adequate nutrition, and preventing complications. However, it's crucial to consult with healthcare professionals or registered dietitians for personalized advice and dietary plans tailored to individual needs and recovery progress.

CHAPTER THREE

Various nutrients play critical roles in maintaining overall health, especially after gastric bypass surgery. Here's an explanation of the importance of specific nutrients:

1. Protein:

• Importance: Essential for tissue repair, muscle maintenance, and immune function.

• Post-Surgery Significance: Vital for healing after surgery and preserving muscle mass during weight loss.

2. Vitamins and Minerals:

a. Vitamin B12:

• Importance: Essential for nerve function, red blood cell production, and DNA synthesis.

• Post-Surgery Significance: Reduced absorption after surgery may lead to deficiencies if not supplemented adequately.

b. Vitamin D:

• Importance: Critical for bone health, calcium absorption, and immune function.

• Post-Surgery Significance: Important due to reduced absorption in the small intestine post-gastric bypass surgery.

c. Iron:

• Importance: Key for red blood cell formation and oxygen transport.

• Post-Surgery Significance: Risk of iron deficiency due to reduced stomach acid and absorption capacity.

d. Calcium:

• Importance: Crucial for bone health, muscle function, and nerve transmission.

• Post-Surgery Significance: Risk of deficiency due to reduced absorption in the smaller stomach pouch.

e. Vitamin A:

• Importance: Supports vision, immune function, and cell growth.

• Post-Surgery Significance: Monitoring necessary due to reduced absorption after surgery.

3. Fiber:

• Importance: Aids in digestion, supports gut health, and helps regulate blood sugar levels.

• Post-Surgery Significance: Gradual reintroduction of fiber-rich foods is important post-surgery to prevent discomfort.

4. Omega-3 Fatty Acids:

• Importance: Supports heart health, brain function, and reduces inflammation.

- Post-Surgery Significance: Important for overall health, especially during weight loss phases.

5. Water and Hydration:

- Importance: Essential for maintaining body temperature, nutrient transportation, and waste elimination.

- Post-Surgery Significance: Crucial for preventing dehydration due to smaller stomach size and reduced liquid intake capacity.

6. Balanced Nutrition:

- Importance: A well-balanced diet provides essential macronutrients (carbohydrates, proteins, fats) and micronutrients (vitamins, minerals) necessary for overall health.

- Post-Surgery Significance: Ensuring a varied and balanced diet supports recovery, prevents deficiencies, and aids in weight management.

After gastric bypass surgery, altered anatomy affects nutrient absorption. Hence, it's crucial to prioritize nutrient-dense foods, follow prescribed supplements, and maintain regular monitoring and follow-up with healthcare professionals to prevent deficiencies and ensure optimal health during the recovery phase and beyond.

Portion control is crucial after gastric bypass surgery due to the reduced stomach size, which limits the amount of food that can be comfortably consumed. Here's the importance of portion control in post-gastric bypass surgery:

1. Adaptation to Smaller Stomach Capacity:

• Limited Capacity: The stomach is significantly reduced in size after surgery, allowing it to hold only a small amount of food at a time.

• Importance: Portion control helps in adjusting to the smaller stomach size, preventing discomfort, nausea, and avoiding stretching of the stomach pouch.

2. Preventing Overeating and Discomfort:

• Avoids Overloading: Smaller portions prevent overwhelming the digestive system and causing discomfort.

• Importance: Eating smaller portions helps in preventing vomiting, nausea, and pain often experienced if larger amounts of food are consumed.

3. Aiding Digestion:

• Easier Digestion: Smaller portions are easier for the reduced stomach size to digest effectively.

• Importance: Properly portioned meals aid in smoother digestion and nutrient absorption, avoiding digestive complications.

4. Weight Management and Weight Loss:

• Controlled Caloric Intake: Portion control assists in managing caloric intake, aiding weight loss efforts.

• Importance: Helps in controlling weight by preventing excessive calorie consumption, promoting gradual and steady weight loss.

5. Preventing Dumping Syndrome:

• Avoidance of Triggers: Controlling portion sizes helps in avoiding foods that may trigger dumping syndrome.

• Importance: Dumping syndrome can cause discomfort, including nausea, sweating, and diarrhea, which can be minimized by portion control and careful food choices.

6. Encouraging Mindful Eating Habits:

• Focus on Satiation: Smaller portions encourage mindfulness about feelings of fullness and satiety.

• Importance: Encourages eating slowly, chewing thoroughly, and paying attention to hunger cues, aiding in better portion control and preventing overeating.

7. Supporting Nutritional Needs:

• Balanced Nutrient Intake: Proper portion control allows for a more balanced intake of nutrients from varied foods.

• Importance: Ensures that the limited space in the stomach is filled with nutrient-dense foods, supporting overall health and preventing deficiencies.

8. Long-Term Habits for Health:

• Cultivating Healthy Eating Patterns: Portion control fosters long-term habits for a healthier lifestyle.

• Importance: Teaches individuals to listen to their bodies, practice moderation, and maintain healthier eating habits for sustained weight management and overall health.

Embracing portion control is fundamental in adapting to the post-gastric bypass anatomy, aiding in proper digestion, supporting weight management, and ensuring adequate nutrition. Consulting with healthcare professionals or registered dietitians for guidance on appropriate portion sizes and meal planning is highly recommended for individuals post-gastric bypass surgery.

THE IMPORTANCE OF HYDRATION

Hydration is crucial for everyone, and particularly so after gastric bypass surgery. Here's why hydration is important post-gastric bypass:

1. Maintaining Fluid Balance:

• Regulates Body Functions: Adequate hydration maintains fluid balance, essential for various bodily functions such as digestion, circulation, and temperature regulation.

2. Prevention of Dehydration:

• Reduced Stomach Capacity: Post-surgery, the stomach's reduced size limits fluid intake at one time.

• Importance: Sipping water throughout the day prevents dehydration, especially when limited fluid intake is a concern.

3. Aid in Digestion and Nutrient Absorption:

• Assists Digestive Processes: Water supports the breakdown of food and the absorption of nutrients.

• Importance: Hydration aids in digestion, ensuring nutrients from the limited food intake are absorbed effectively.

4. Prevention of Constipation:

• Common Post-Surgery Issue: Constipation can occur due to changes in diet and reduced fiber intake.

• Importance: Proper hydration softens stools and prevents constipation, promoting regular bowel movements.

5. Facilitation of Healing and Recovery:

• Supports Healing Processes: Hydration is essential for tissue repair and wound healing.

• Importance: Optimal hydration aids in the body's recovery process after surgery.

6. Regulation of Body Temperature:

• Assists in Temperature Control: Adequate hydration helps regulate body temperature, especially during physical activity or in warmer climates.

7. Prevention of Complications:

• Reduces Risks: Adequate hydration minimizes the risks of urinary tract infections and kidney stones.

• Importance: Helps in preventing potential complications associated with dehydration.

8. Supports Overall Health:

• Promotes General Wellness: Hydration is crucial for overall health, including skin health, joint lubrication, and cognitive function.

Tips for Hydration after Gastric Bypass Surgery:

• Sip Water Throughout the Day: Drinking small amounts of water between meals helps maintain hydration without overloading the stomach.

• Avoid Drinking with Meals: Limiting fluids during meals prevents discomfort and allows for better digestion.

• Monitor Urine Color: Light-colored urine indicates good hydration, while dark-colored urine may indicate dehydration.

• Include Hydrating Foods: Consume hydrating foods like fruits and vegetables with high water content to supplement hydration needs.

Maintaining adequate hydration after gastric bypass surgery is vital for supporting recovery, preventing complications, and ensuring overall well-being. Individuals should follow personalized hydration guidelines provided by healthcare professionals or registered dietitians to meet their specific needs post-surgery.

Following gastric bypass surgery, several challenges might arise related to dietary changes. These challenges can vary among individuals, but common ones include:

1. Adjusting to New Eating Patterns:

• Limited Stomach Capacity: Adjusting to smaller portion sizes and reduced food intake capacity can be challenging.

• Impact: Individuals may feel unsatisfied after smaller meals initially, requiring time to adapt to new eating habits.

2. Meeting Nutritional Needs:

• Risk of Nutrient Deficiencies: Difficulty in meeting nutritional needs due to reduced food intake and altered absorption.

• Impact: Risk of deficiencies in vitamins (B12, D, A, etc.) and minerals (iron, calcium) if not supplemented adequately.

3. Reintroducing Foods Gradually:

• Progressive Diet Phases: Gradual reintroduction of foods in stages as advised by healthcare professionals.

• Impact: Adhering to specific diet stages (liquids, purees, soft foods) can be challenging, requiring patience and compliance.

4. Hydration Challenges:

• Fluid Intake Adjustments: Learning to sip water throughout the day between meals instead of drinking large amounts at once.

• Impact: Ensuring adequate hydration without causing discomfort or exceeding the stomach's capacity.

5. Identifying Trigger Foods:

• Avoidance of Certain Foods: Identifying and avoiding foods that cause discomfort, dumping syndrome, or digestive issues.

• Impact: Requires trial and error to determine foods that are well-tolerated and those that should be avoided post-surgery.

6. Developing New Eating Habits:

• Mindful Eating Practices: Adopting mindful eating habits, chewing food thoroughly, and eating slowly.

• Impact: Learning new eating behaviors and paying attention to hunger and satiety cues can be challenging but essential for success.

7. Emotional and Psychological Adjustments:

• Emotional Eating: Coping with emotional triggers that might lead to overeating or unhealthy food choices.

• Impact: Addressing emotional eating patterns and seeking support to manage emotional aspects of dietary changes.

8. Social and Lifestyle Adjustments:

• Social Situations: Adjusting to social gatherings and events where food choices might be challenging or tempting.

• Impact: Learning to navigate social settings while adhering to dietary guidelines without feeling isolated.

9. Long-Term Maintenance:

• Sustaining Lifestyle Changes: Maintaining dietary modifications and healthy habits for the long term.

• Impact: Requires ongoing commitment, support, and motivation to ensure continued success and prevent weight regain.

Addressing these challenges requires patience, perseverance, and support from healthcare professionals, dietitians, support groups, and loved ones. Understanding and managing these challenges can significantly contribute to successful recovery and long-term success post-gastric bypass surgery.

PRACTICAL COOKING ADVICE

Here are some practical cooking tips that can be helpful for individuals post-gastric bypass surgery or anyone looking to prepare nutritious meals:

1. Prioritize Nutrient-Dense Ingredients:

• Choose Whole Foods: Opt for fresh fruits, vegetables, lean proteins (chicken, fish, tofu), whole grains, and healthy fats (avocado, nuts) to ensure a balanced and nutritious diet.

2. Portion Control and Meal Prepping:

• Pre-Portion Ingredients: Portion out ingredients in advance to control serving sizes and prevent overeating.

• Meal Prep: Prepare meals in advance to have healthy options readily available, making it easier to stick to dietary goals.

3. Opt for Healthier Cooking Methods:

• Grilling, Baking, Steaming: Use cooking techniques that require less fat or oil to reduce unnecessary calories while preserving flavor.

• Avoid Frying: Minimize deep-frying or pan-frying to limit added fats.

4. Experiment with Herbs and Spices:

• Flavorful Alternatives: Use herbs, spices, citrus, and vinegar to add flavor to dishes without relying on excess salt, sugar, or fat.

• Be Creative: Experiment with different combinations to enhance taste without compromising on healthiness.

5. Read Food Labels:

• Check Nutritional Information: Pay attention to labels for portion sizes, calorie content, sugar, and fat to make informed choices when purchasing packaged foods.

6. Mindful Cooking and Eating:

• Chew Thoroughly: Encourage mindful eating by chewing food slowly and thoroughly, aiding digestion and preventing discomfort.

• Eat Mindfully: Enjoy meals without distractions, focusing on hunger cues and stopping when satisfied.

7. Hydration and Healthy Beverages:

• Water Intake: Ensure regular hydration by drinking water throughout the day. Infuse water with fruits or herbs for added flavor.

• Limit Sugary Drinks: Avoid high-sugar beverages and opt for healthier choices like herbal teas, infused water, or low-calorie options.

8. Adapt Recipes to Dietary Needs:

• Customize Recipes: Modify recipes to fit dietary requirements, such as using low-fat ingredients or swapping out ingredients to reduce sugar content.

9. Use Small Kitchen Tools:

• Portion-Sized Utensils: Use smaller plates, bowls, and utensils to visually manage portion sizes and prevent overeating.

10. Seek Support and Resources:

• Join Support Groups: Connect with others who have undergone similar experiences or seek advice from nutritionists, dietitians, or online communities for meal ideas and support.

Practicing these cooking tips can contribute to a more enjoyable and healthier culinary experience post-gastric bypass surgery or when aiming for a balanced diet and lifestyle. It's essential to tailor cooking habits to individual dietary needs and preferences while maintaining a focus on nutrition and portion control.

INGREDIENTS SUBSTITUTIONS

Ingredient substitutions involve replacing one ingredient in a recipe with another due to dietary restrictions, preferences, allergies, or ingredient availability. Here are some common ingredient substitutions:

1. Flour:

• Whole Wheat Flour: Can often substitute for all-purpose flour in many recipes, offering more fiber and nutrients.

• Gluten-Free Flours (Almond, Coconut, Oat): Suitable for those with gluten intolerance or celiac disease.

2. Sugar:

• Natural Sweeteners (Stevia, Monk Fruit, Erythritol): Lower-calorie alternatives for those seeking to reduce sugar intake.

• Maple Syrup, Honey, or Agave Nectar: Can substitute refined sugar, adding a different flavor profile.

3. Butter/Oil:

• Applesauce or Mashed Banana: Use in baking recipes as a replacement for part or all of the butter or oil to reduce fat content.

• Greek Yogurt: Substituted for oil or butter in some recipes to lower fat content while maintaining moisture.

4. Milk/Dairy:

• Almond, Soy, Coconut, or Oat Milk: Substitutes for cow's milk, suitable for lactose intolerance or vegan diets.

• Yogurt or Buttermilk: Substitutes for heavy cream in savory dishes or baking.

5. Eggs:

• Flaxseeds or Chia Seeds: Mixed with water to create a gel-like consistency as an egg substitute in baking.

• Silken Tofu or Applesauce: Used in recipes that require binding or moisture.

6. Salt:

• Herbs, Spices, and Vinegar: Substitute for salt to add flavor without sodium.

7. Meat:

• Tofu, Tempeh, Seitan: Substitutes for meat in vegetarian or vegan recipes.

• Mushrooms or Lentils: Used to add texture and flavor similar to ground meat in dishes like burgers or sauces.

Tips for Successful Substitutions:

• Consider Flavor Profiles: Ensure the substitute complements the dish's overall taste and doesn't overpower other ingredients.

• Be Mindful of Textures: Some substitutions may alter the texture of the final dish, so adjust accordingly.

• Follow Ratios: Substitute ingredients in proper ratios to maintain the recipe's balance and consistency.

• Experiment and Taste: Try small batches or adjustments first to ensure the substitution works well before preparing the entire recipe.

When substituting ingredients, especially in baking, it's essential to be cautious as certain changes may affect the final taste, texture, or overall outcome of the dish. It's recommended to gradually introduce substitutions and adjust quantities to suit personal preferences while maintaining the dish's integrity.

TIPS AND ADVICE FOR MAINTAINING A HEALTHY LIFESTYLE AND ACHIEVING LONG-TERM SUCCESS AFTER SURGERY.

Maintaining a healthy lifestyle and achieving long-term success after surgery, such as gastric bypass, involves a holistic approach focusing on diet, exercise, mental well-being, and consistent habits. Here are practical tips and strategies:

1. Follow Post-Surgery Guidelines:

• Adhere to Medical Advice: Follow the post-operative instructions provided by healthcare professionals regarding diet progression, physical activity, and follow-up appointments.

2. Balanced Nutrition:

• Healthy Eating Habits: Embrace a balanced diet rich in lean proteins, vegetables, fruits, whole grains, and healthy fats while monitoring portion sizes.

• Nutritional Supplements: Take prescribed vitamins and minerals to prevent deficiencies.

3. Regular Exercise:

• Gradual Activity Increase: Begin with low-impact exercises and gradually progress to more intense workouts as advised by healthcare providers.

• Consistency is Key: Establish a regular exercise routine focusing on both cardiovascular workouts and strength training for overall fitness.

4. Mindful Eating Practices:

• Eat Slowly and Chew Thoroughly: Practice mindful eating to aid digestion, prevent discomfort, and recognize feelings of fullness.

• Avoid Distractions: Minimize distractions during meals to focus on eating and recognize satiety cues.

5. Stay Hydrated:

• Fluid Intake: Drink water throughout the day between meals, prioritizing hydration without consuming excessive fluids during meals.

6. Emotional Well-being:

• Address Emotional Triggers: Develop coping mechanisms for managing stress, emotions, and potential triggers for emotional eating.

• Seek Support: Consider therapy, support groups, or counseling to navigate emotional aspects of the journey.

7. Regular Follow-ups:

• Scheduled Check-ups: Attend follow-up appointments with healthcare professionals, including dietitians, to monitor progress and address any concerns.

8. Behavioral Changes:

• Establish Healthy Habits: Create sustainable lifestyle changes, focusing on long-term health goals rather than short-term fixes.

• Track Progress: Keep a food diary, record exercise routines, and monitor weight changes to track progress and stay accountable.

9. Social Support and Community Engagement:

• Join Support Groups: Connect with others who have undergone similar experiences for advice, encouragement, and sharing experiences.

• Involve Loved Ones: Educate family and friends about your journey to receive support and encouragement.

10. Celebrate Non-Scale Victories:

• Acknowledge Achievements: Celebrate milestones beyond weight loss, such as increased energy levels, improved fitness, or healthier habits.

11. Stay Informed and Educated:

• Continual Learning: Stay updated on nutrition, exercise, and health-related information to make informed choices.

12. Patience and Perseverance:

• Realistic Expectations: Understand that progress may take time, and setbacks can occur. Be patient and stay committed to the long-term goal.

Maintaining a healthy lifestyle after surgery requires dedication, commitment, and a holistic approach encompassing physical, nutritional, and mental well-being. Consistency, patience, and seeking support from healthcare professionals and a supportive community play vital roles in achieving long-term success.

CHAPTER FOUR

BREAKFAST RECIPES

Greek Yogurt Parfait

Ingredients:

• 1/2 cup Greek yogurt (low-fat or non-fat)

• 1/4 cup fresh berries (strawberries, blueberries, or raspberries)

• 1 tablespoon chopped nuts (almonds, walnuts)

• 1 teaspoon honey or maple syrup (optional for added sweetness)

Instructions:

1. In a small bowl or glass, layer half of the Greek yogurt. Add half of the berries on top of the yogurt layer.

2. Sprinkle half of the chopped nuts over the berries. Repeat the layers with the remaining yogurt, berries, and nuts.

3. Drizzle honey or maple syrup over the top if desired.

4. Enjoy this protein-packed parfait with a small spoon, eating slowly and savoring each bite.

Ingredients:

- 2 large eggs

- 1/4 cup chopped spinach

- 2 tablespoons crumbled feta cheese

- Salt and pepper to taste

Instructions:

1. Preheat oven to 350°F (175°C). Grease a muffin tin or use silicone muffin cups.

2. In a bowl, beat the eggs and season with salt and pepper. Divide the chopped spinach and feta evenly among the muffin cups.

3. Pour the beaten eggs into each cup, filling them about 3/4 full. Bake for 15-20 minutes or until the egg muffins are set and slightly golden.

4. Allow them to cool slightly before removing from the muffin tin.

5. Serve warm and enjoy a protein-packed breakfast option.

Overnight Chia Seed Pudding

Ingredients:

- 2 tablespoons chia seeds

- 1/2 cup unsweetened almond milk (or any preferred milk)

- 1/4 teaspoon vanilla extract

- 1/4 cup diced fruits (such as mangoes, peaches, or kiwi)

- 1 tablespoon shredded coconut (optional)

Instructions:

1. In a small jar or bowl, mix the chia seeds, almond milk, and vanilla extract.

2. Stir well to ensure the chia seeds are evenly distributed in the milk. Cover the jar/bowl and refrigerate overnight or for at least 4 hours.

3. Before serving, stir the mixture to break up any clumps that may have formed.

4. Top with diced fruits and shredded coconut for added flavor and texture.

5. Enjoy this fiber-rich pudding with a small spoon.

Cottage Cheese Pancakes

Ingredients:

- 1/2 cup cottage cheese (low-fat or non-fat)

- 2 tablespoons oat flour or almond flour

- 1 egg

- 1/4 teaspoon baking powder

- 1/4 teaspoon vanilla extract

- Berries or sliced fruit for topping (optional)

Instructions:

1. In a blender or mixing bowl, combine cottage cheese, oat/almond flour, egg, baking powder, and vanilla extract. Blend or mix until smooth.

2. Heat a non-stick skillet or griddle over medium heat and lightly grease with cooking spray or a small amount of oil.

3. Pour small portions of the batter onto the skillet to form pancakes (about 2-3 inches in diameter).

4. Cook for 2-3 minutes on each side or until golden brown. Top with berries or sliced fruit if desired.

5. Serve warm and enjoy these protein-packed pancakes.

Avocado and Egg Breakfast Bowl

Ingredients:

• 1 small ripe avocado

• 1 hard-boiled egg, sliced

• Dash of lime juice

• Salt, pepper, and paprika to taste

• Fresh herbs for garnish (optional)

Instructions:

1. Cut the avocado in half, remove the pit, and scoop a little extra flesh from each half to create space for the egg.

2. Sprinkle the avocado halves with a dash of lime juice, salt, pepper, and paprika.

3. Carefully place the sliced hard-boiled egg inside each avocado half.

4. Garnish with fresh herbs if desired.

Veggie Omelette

Ingredients:

• 2 eggs

• 1/4 cup diced bell peppers

- 1/4 cup diced tomatoes

- 1 tablespoon diced onions

- 1 tablespoon chopped spinach

- 1 tablespoon shredded cheese (optional)

- Salt and pepper to taste

Instructions:

1. In a bowl, beat the eggs and season with salt and pepper.

2. Heat a non-stick skillet over medium heat and lightly grease it with cooking spray or a small amount of oil.

3. Pour the beaten eggs into the skillet.

4. Sprinkle the diced bell peppers, tomatoes, onions, spinach, and shredded cheese evenly over one half of the cooking eggs.

5. Once the eggs are mostly set, carefully fold the omelette in half. Cook for an additional minute or until the cheese (if using) melts.

6. Slide the omelette onto a plate and serve warm.

Banana Almond Butter Toast

Ingredients:

• 1 slice whole-grain or multigrain bread

• 1 tablespoon almond butter

• 1/2 ripe banana, thinly sliced

• Cinnamon (optional)

Instructions:

1. Toast the bread to your desired level of crispiness. Spread the almond butter evenly on the toasted bread slice.

2. Arrange the thinly sliced banana on top of the almond butter.

3. Sprinkle a pinch of cinnamon for added flavor if desired.

4. Enjoy this simple and satisfying breakfast toast.

Protein-Packed Smoothie Bowl

Ingredients:

• 1/2 cup Greek yogurt (low-fat or non-fat)

• 1/2 frozen banana

• 1/4 cup frozen berries (such as strawberries, blueberries)

• 1 tablespoon chia seeds or flaxseeds

• Toppings: Sliced fruits, nuts, seeds, or shredded coconut (optional)

Instructions:

1. In a blender, combine the Greek yogurt, frozen banana, frozen berries, and chia seeds.

2. Blend until smooth and creamy, adding a splash of water or milk if needed to reach the desired consistency.

3. Pour the smoothie into a bowl.

4. Top with sliced fruits, nuts, seeds, or shredded coconut for added texture and nutrients.

5. Enjoy this protein-rich smoothie bowl with a spoon.

Ricotta and Berries Breakfast Bowl

Ingredients:

• 1/4 cup part-skim ricotta cheese

• 1/4 cup mixed berries (such as raspberries, blueberries)

• 1 tablespoon chopped nuts (such as almonds, walnuts)

• 1 teaspoon honey (optional for added sweetness)

Instructions:

1. In a small bowl, spoon the ricotta cheese. Top the ricotta with mixed berries and chopped nuts.

2. Drizzle honey over the top if desired for a touch of sweetness.

3. Mix gently and enjoy this creamy and nutritious breakfast bowl.

Quinoa Breakfast Porridge

Ingredients:

- 1/4 cup cooked quinoa

- 1/4 cup unsweetened almond milk (or any preferred milk)

- 1 tablespoon chopped nuts (such as pecans, almonds)

- 1 tablespoon dried fruits (such as cranberries, raisins)

- Cinnamon or nutmeg for flavor (optional)

Instructions:

1. In a small saucepan, warm the cooked quinoa with almond milk over medium-low heat.

2. Stir in chopped nuts, dried fruits, and a pinch of cinnamon or nutmeg if desired.

3. Cook for a few minutes until heated through and the porridge reaches the desired consistency.

4. Transfer to a bowl and enjoy this hearty and fiber-rich quinoa porridge.

Ingredients:

- 1/4 cup rolled oats

- 1/3 cup unsweetened almond milk (or any preferred milk)

- 1/4 cup grated apple

- 1 tablespoon chopped nuts (such as walnuts or almonds)

- 1/2 teaspoon cinnamon

- 1 teaspoon honey or maple syrup (optional for added sweetness)

Instructions:

1. In a jar or bowl, combine rolled oats, almond milk, grated apple, chopped nuts, cinnamon, and honey/maple syrup if desired.

2. Stir well to mix all ingredients thoroughly. Cover the jar or bowl and refrigerate overnight or for at least 4 hours.

3. Before serving, give it a good stir and add a little extra almond milk if preferred.

4. Enjoy this fiber-packed and delicious breakfast option.

Ingredients:

• 1 whole wheat or corn tortilla

• 1 egg, scrambled

• 1/4 cup diced bell peppers

• 1/4 cup chopped spinach

• 1 tablespoon shredded cheese (optional)

• Salt and pepper to taste

Instructions:

1. In a skillet over medium heat, lightly cook the diced bell peppers and chopped spinach until softened.

2. Add the scrambled egg to the skillet and cook until done.

3. Warm the tortilla in the microwave or on a separate skillet for a few seconds.

4. Place the cooked egg, vegetables, and shredded cheese (if using) in the center of the tortilla. Fold the sides of the tortilla towards the center, creating a wrap.

5. Enjoy this protein-packed breakfast wrap.

Turkey and Veggie Breakfast Skewers

Ingredients:

- 2 oz turkey breast slices

- 1/4 cup cherry tomatoes

- 1/4 cup cucumber slices

- 1/4 cup bell pepper chunks

- Wooden skewers

Instructions:

1. Thread the turkey slices, cherry tomatoes, cucumber slices, and bell pepper chunks onto wooden skewers in an alternating pattern.

2. Heat a grill pan or non-stick skillet over medium-high heat.

3. Cook the skewers for a few minutes on each side until the turkey is cooked through and vegetables are slightly charred.

4. Serve these protein-packed skewers for a flavorful and satisfying breakfast.

Almond Flour Banana Muffins

Ingredients:

- 1 cup almond flour

- 1 ripe banana, mashed

- 2 eggs

- 1 tablespoon honey or maple syrup

- 1/4 teaspoon baking soda

- 1/4 teaspoon vanilla extract

Instructions:

1. Preheat oven to 350°F (175°C). Line a muffin tin with liners or grease it lightly.

2. In a bowl, mix together almond flour, mashed banana, eggs, honey/maple syrup, baking soda, and vanilla extract until well combined.

3. Divide the batter evenly into muffin cups, filling them about 3/4 full.

4. Bake for 18-20 minutes or until a toothpick inserted into the center comes out clean.

5. Allow the muffins to cool in the pan for a few minutes before transferring to a wire rack.

6. Enjoy these gluten-free almond flour banana muffins as a delightful breakfast option.

Protein-Packed Breakfast Burrito Bowl

Ingredients:

• 1/4 cup cooked quinoa or brown rice

• 1/4 cup black beans, drained and rinsed

• 1 scrambled egg

• 2 tablespoons salsa

• 1 tablespoon chopped avocado

• Fresh cilantro for garnish (optional)

Instructions:

1. In a bowl, layer cooked quinoa/brown rice, black beans, and scrambled egg.

2. Top with salsa and chopped avocado. Garnish with fresh cilantro if desired.

3. Enjoy this protein and fiber-rich breakfast burrito bowl.

Veggie Breakfast Quiche Cups

Ingredients:

• 2 eggs

• 1/4 cup diced bell peppers

• 1/4 cup chopped spinach

- 1 tablespoon diced onions

- 2 tablespoons shredded cheese (optional)

- Salt and pepper to taste

Instructions:

1. Preheat the oven to 350°F (175°C). Grease a muffin tin or use silicone muffin cups.

2. In a bowl, whisk the eggs and season with salt and pepper.

3. Divide the diced bell peppers, chopped spinach, onions, and shredded cheese (if using) evenly among the muffin cups.

4. Pour the whisked eggs into each cup, filling them about 3/4 full. Bake for 15-20 minutes or until the quiche cups are set and slightly golden.

5. Allow them to cool slightly before removing from the muffin tin.

6. Serve warm and enjoy these protein-packed quiche cups.

Peanut Butter Banana Smoothie

Ingredients:

- 1/2 ripe banana

- 1 tablespoon natural peanut butter

- 1/2 cup unsweetened almond milk (or any preferred milk)

- 1 tablespoon Greek yogurt (low-fat or non-fat)

- 1 teaspoon honey (optional for added sweetness)

- Ice cubes (optional)

Instructions:

1. In a blender, combine the ripe banana, peanut butter, almond milk, Greek yogurt, and honey if using.

2. Add a few ice cubes if desired for a colder texture. Blend until smooth and creamy.

3. Pour the smoothie into a glass and enjoy this protein-rich beverage.

Ricotta and Berry Pancakes

Ingredients:

- 1/4 cup part-skim ricotta cheese

- 1 egg

- 2 tablespoons oat flour or almond flour

- 1/4 teaspoon baking powder

- 1/4 cup mixed berries (such as blueberries, raspberries)

- Cooking spray or a small amount of oil for greasing

Instructions:

1. In a bowl, whisk together ricotta cheese, egg, oat/almond flour, and baking powder until well combined.

2. Gently fold in the mixed berries into the batter.

3. Heat a non-stick skillet or griddle over medium heat and lightly grease it.

4. Pour small portions of the batter onto the skillet to form pancakes. Cook for 2-3 minutes on each side or until golden brown.

5. Serve warm and enjoy these protein-packed pancakes with a touch of sweetness from the berries.

Turkey and Egg Breakfast Cups

Ingredients:

• 2 oz turkey breast slices

• 2 eggs

• 1/4 cup diced tomatoes

• 1 tablespoon chopped spinach

• Salt and pepper to taste

Instructions:

1. Preheat the oven to 350°F (175°C). Grease a muffin tin or use silicone muffin cups.

2. Line each cup with turkey slices to create a cup shape. Crack an egg into each turkey cup.

3. Sprinkle diced tomatoes, chopped spinach, salt, and pepper on top. Bake for 15-18 minutes or until the eggs are set.

4. Allow them to cool slightly before removing from the muffin tin.

5. Serve warm and enjoy these protein-packed breakfast cups.

Cottage Cheese and Fruit Bowl

Ingredients:

• 1/2 cup cottage cheese (low-fat or non-fat)

• 1/4 cup diced fruits (such as pineapple, mango, or peaches)

• 1 tablespoon chopped nuts (such as almonds or walnuts)

• 1 teaspoon honey or maple syrup (optional for added sweetness)

Instructions:

1. In a bowl, spoon the cottage cheese.

2. Top with diced fruits and chopped nuts. Drizzle honey or maple syrup for a touch of sweetness if desired.

3. Mix gently and enjoy this protein-rich and fruity breakfast bowl.

Veggie and Cheese Frittata Cups

Ingredients:

• 2 eggs

• 2 tablespoons diced bell peppers

• 2 tablespoons chopped spinach

• 2 tablespoons diced tomatoes

• 2 tablespoons shredded cheese (optional)

• Salt and pepper to taste

Instructions:

1. Preheat the oven to 350°F (175°C). Grease a muffin tin or use silicone muffin cups.

2. In a bowl, whisk the eggs and season with salt and pepper.

3. Divide the diced bell peppers, chopped spinach, diced tomatoes, and shredded cheese (if using) among the muffin cups.

4. Pour the whisked eggs evenly into each cup, filling them about 3/4 full. Bake for 15-18 minutes or until the frittata cups are set and slightly golden.

5. Allow them to cool slightly before removing from the muffin tin.

6. Serve warm and enjoy these veggie-packed frittata cups.

Berry and Yogurt Breakfast Bowl

Ingredients:

• 1/2 cup Greek yogurt (low-fat or non-fat)

• 1/4 cup mixed berries (such as strawberries, blueberries)

• 1 tablespoon chopped nuts (such as almonds or walnuts)

• 1 teaspoon honey or maple syrup (optional for added sweetness)

Instructions:

1. In a bowl, spoon the Greek yogurt.

2. Top with mixed berries and chopped nuts. Drizzle honey or maple syrup for a touch of sweetness if desired.

3. Mix gently and enjoy this protein-rich and fruity breakfast bowl.

Ingredients:

• 1 slice whole-grain or multigrain bread

• 2 oz smoked salmon

• 1/4 ripe avocado, thinly sliced

• Lemon juice (optional)

• Fresh dill or chives for garnish (optional)

Instructions:

1. Toast the bread to your desired level of crispiness. Spread the thinly sliced avocado on the toasted bread.

2. Layer smoked salmon on top of the avocado. Squeeze a little lemon juice over the salmon for added freshness if desired.

3. Garnish with fresh dill or chives if available.

4. Enjoy this flavorful and protein-rich smoked salmon and avocado toast.

Spinach and Mushroom Egg Muffins

Ingredients:

• 2 eggs

• 1/4 cup chopped spinach

- 2 tablespoons diced mushrooms

- 1 tablespoon diced onions

- Salt and pepper to taste

Instructions:

1. Preheat the oven to 350°F (175°C). Grease a muffin tin or use silicone muffin cups.

2. In a bowl, beat the eggs and season with salt and pepper.

3. Divide the chopped spinach, diced mushrooms, and diced onions evenly among the muffin cups.

4. Pour the beaten eggs into each cup, filling them about 3/4 full. Bake for 15-18 minutes or until the egg muffins are set and slightly golden.

5. Allow them to cool slightly before removing from the muffin tin.

6. Serve warm and enjoy these veggie-packed egg muffins.

Berry and Almond Milk Smoothie

Ingredients:

- 1/2 cup unsweetened almond milk (or any preferred milk)

- 1/2 cup mixed berries (such as raspberries, blackberries)

- 1 tablespoon almond butter

• 1 tablespoon Greek yogurt (low-fat or non-fat)

• Ice cubes (optional)

Instructions:

1. In a blender, combine almond milk, mixed berries, almond butter, and Greek yogurt.

2. Add a few ice cubes if desired for a colder texture.

3. Blend until smooth and creamy.

4. Pour the smoothie into a glass and enjoy this antioxidant-rich beverage.

Banana Walnut Breakfast Cookies

Ingredients:

• 1 ripe banana, mashed

• 1/2 cup rolled oats

• 2 tablespoons chopped walnuts

• 1 tablespoon unsweetened applesauce

• 1 tablespoon honey or maple syrup (optional)

• 1/4 teaspoon cinnamon

• Pinch of salt

Instructions:

1. Preheat the oven to 350°F (175°C). Line a baking sheet with parchment paper.

2. In a bowl, mix mashed banana, rolled oats, chopped walnuts, applesauce, honey/maple syrup (if using), cinnamon, and a pinch of salt until well combined.

3. Spoon the mixture onto the baking sheet, forming small cookie shapes.

4. Bake for 15-18 minutes or until lightly golden.

5. Allow the cookies to cool on the baking sheet before serving.

Caprese Egg Muffins

Ingredients:

- 2 eggs

- 1/4 cup diced tomatoes

- 2 tablespoons chopped fresh basil

- 2 tablespoons shredded mozzarella cheese

- Salt and pepper to taste

Instructions:

1. Preheat the oven to 350°F (175°C). Grease a muffin tin or use silicone muffin cups.

2. In a bowl, beat the eggs and season with salt and pepper.

3. Divide the diced tomatoes, chopped fresh basil, and shredded mozzarella evenly among the muffin cups.

4. Pour the beaten eggs into each cup, filling them about 3/4 full. Bake for 15-18 minutes or until the egg muffins are set.

5. Allow them to cool slightly before removing from the muffin tin.

6. Serve warm and enjoy these flavorful Caprese egg muffins.

Green Smoothie Bowl

Ingredients:

• 1/2 ripe avocado

• 1/2 cup spinach leaves

• 1/2 cup unsweetened almond milk (or any preferred milk)

• 1/2 frozen banana

• Toppings: Sliced fruits, nuts, seeds, or shredded coconut (optional)

Instructions:

1. In a blender, combine avocado, spinach leaves, almond milk, and frozen banana.

2. Blend until smooth and creamy, adding a splash of water or more milk if needed for desired consistency.

3. Pour the smoothie into a bowl. Top with sliced fruits, nuts, seeds, or shredded coconut for added texture and nutrients.

4. Enjoy this nutrient-packed green smoothie bowl with a spoon.

Turkey and Veggie Breakfast Skillet

Ingredients:

• 2 oz turkey sausage or turkey bacon, diced

• 1/4 cup diced bell peppers

• 1/4 cup diced zucchini

• 1/4 cup diced onions

• 2 eggs

• Salt and pepper to taste

Instructions:

1. In a skillet over medium heat, cook the diced turkey sausage or turkey bacon until slightly browned.

2. Add diced bell peppers, zucchini, and onions to the skillet. Sauté until vegetables are tender.

3. Crack the eggs into the skillet, seasoning with salt and pepper.

4. Cook until the eggs are done to your liking.

5. Serve warm and enjoy this protein and veggie-rich breakfast skillet.

Chia Seed Pudding with Berries

Ingredients:

• 2 tablespoons chia seeds

• 1/2 cup unsweetened almond milk (or any preferred milk)

• 1/4 teaspoon vanilla extract

• 1/4 cup mixed berries (such as strawberries, blueberries)

• 1 tablespoon chopped nuts (such as almonds or pecans)

Instructions:

1. In a bowl or jar, mix chia seeds, almond milk, and vanilla extract. Stir well to combine.

2. Refrigerate the mixture for at least 2 hours or overnight until it thickens.

3. Before serving, stir the pudding to ensure it's well combined. Top with mixed berries and chopped nuts.

4. Enjoy this fiber-rich chia seed pudding with delightful berries.

Quinoa and Veggie Salad

Ingredients:

- 1/2 cup cooked quinoa

- 1/4 cup diced cucumber

- 1/4 cup diced bell peppers (assorted colors)

- 2 tablespoons diced tomatoes

- 2 tablespoons chopped fresh parsley

- 1 tablespoon lemon juice

- 1 tablespoon olive oil

- Salt and pepper to taste

Instructions:

1. In a bowl, combine cooked quinoa, diced cucumber, bell peppers, tomatoes, and fresh parsley.

2. Drizzle lemon juice and olive oil over the mixture.

3. Season with salt and pepper according to taste. Toss gently until well combined.

4. Serve immediately or refrigerate for a few hours before enjoying this refreshing quinoa and veggie salad.

Ingredients:

- 4 large lettuce leaves (such as romaine or iceberg)

- 4 oz cooked turkey breast, shredded

- 1/4 cup diced tomatoes

- 2 tablespoons diced bell peppers

- 2 tablespoons diced onions

- 2 tablespoons hummus or Greek yogurt (as a spread)

- Fresh herbs for garnish (optional)

Instructions:

1. Lay out the lettuce leaves on a clean surface.

2. Spread hummus or Greek yogurt on each lettuce leaf.

3. Divide shredded turkey, diced tomatoes, bell peppers, and onions evenly among the lettuce leaves. Garnish with fresh herbs if desired.

4. Roll up the lettuce leaves to form wraps and secure with toothpicks if necessary.

5. Serve these turkey lettuce wraps as a light and satisfying lunch option.

Ingredients:

- 3 oz grilled or baked salmon fillet, flaked

- 1/4 avocado, sliced

- 2 cups mixed greens (such as spinach, arugula)

- 1/4 cup cucumber slices

- 1/4 cup cherry tomatoes, halved

- 1 tablespoon olive oil

- 1 tablespoon balsamic vinegar

- Salt and pepper to taste

Instructions:

1. In a large bowl, combine mixed greens, cucumber slices, and cherry tomatoes.

2. Top with flaked salmon and sliced avocado. Drizzle olive oil and balsamic vinegar over the salad.

3. Season with salt and pepper according to taste. Gently toss the salad until ingredients are well coated.

4. Enjoy this flavorful and nutritious salmon and avocado salad.

Ingredients:

- 4 oz cooked chicken breast, sliced

- 1/2 cup broccoli florets

- 1/2 cup sliced bell peppers (assorted colors)

- 1/4 cup sliced carrots

- 1/4 cup sliced mushrooms

- 2 tablespoons low-sodium soy sauce or tamari

- 1 tablespoon olive oil

- 1 teaspoon minced garlic

- 1/2 teaspoon grated ginger (optional)

Instructions:

1. Heat olive oil in a skillet or wok over medium-high heat.

2. Add minced garlic and grated ginger (if using), sautéing for a minute. Add sliced chicken breast and stir-fry for 2-3 minutes until heated through.

3. Add broccoli florets, sliced bell peppers, carrots, and mushrooms to the skillet. Stir-fry for an additional 4-5 minutes until the vegetables are tender yet crisp.

4. Pour low-sodium soy sauce or tamari over the stir-fry and toss to combine.

5. Serve this colorful and nutritious veggie and chicken stir-fry immediately.

Tuna and White Bean Salad

Ingredients:

• 1 can (5 oz) tuna in water, drained

• 1/2 cup canned white beans, drained and rinsed

• 2 cups mixed greens (such as lettuce, spinach)

• 2 tablespoons diced red onions

• 1 tablespoon chopped fresh parsley

• 1 tablespoon lemon juice

• 1 tablespoon olive oil

• Salt and pepper to taste

Instructions:

1. In a bowl, combine drained tuna, white beans, mixed greens, diced red onions, and chopped parsley.

2. Drizzle lemon juice and olive oil over the salad. Season with salt and pepper according to taste.

3. Gently toss the salad until ingredients are well mixed.

4. Serve this protein-packed tuna and white bean salad for a satisfying lunch.

Veggie Egg Salad Lettuce Wraps

Ingredients:

• 2 hard-boiled eggs, chopped

• 1/4 cup diced cucumbers

• 1/4 cup diced bell peppers (assorted colors)

• 2 tablespoons diced red onions

• 2 tablespoons Greek yogurt (low-fat or non-fat)

• 1 teaspoon Dijon mustard

• Salt and pepper to taste

• 4 large lettuce leaves (such as romaine or butter lettuce)

Instructions:

1. In a bowl, combine chopped hard-boiled eggs, diced cucumbers, bell peppers, and red onions.

2. Add Greek yogurt, Dijon mustard, salt, and pepper to the mixture. Mix well.

3. Lay out the lettuce leaves on a clean surface. Spoon the egg salad mixture onto each lettuce leaf.

4. Wrap the lettuce leaves around the filling to form wraps. Secure with toothpicks if necessary.

5. Serve these refreshing and protein-rich veggie egg salad wraps.

Grilled Chicken and Veggie Skewers

Ingredients:

• 4 oz chicken breast, cut into cubes

• 1/2 cup cherry tomatoes

• 1/2 cup bell pepper chunks (assorted colors)

• 1/2 cup zucchini chunks

• 1 tablespoon olive oil

• 1 teaspoon minced garlic

• Salt and pepper to taste

• Wooden skewers

Instructions:

1. Preheat a grill or grill pan over medium-high heat.

2. Thread chicken cubes, cherry tomatoes, bell pepper chunks, and zucchini chunks onto wooden skewers in an alternating pattern.

3. In a small bowl, mix olive oil, minced garlic, salt, and pepper. Brush the skewers with the olive oil mixture.

4. Grill the skewers for 8-10 minutes, turning occasionally, until the chicken is cooked through and the veggies are slightly charred.

5. Serve these flavorful grilled chicken and veggie skewers as a delicious and protein-packed lunch option.

Lentil and Vegetable Soup

Ingredients:

- 1/2 cup cooked lentils

- 2 cups low-sodium vegetable broth

- 1/4 cup diced carrots

- 1/4 cup diced celery

- 1/4 cup diced onions

- 1 teaspoon olive oil

- 1/2 teaspoon dried thyme

- Salt and pepper to taste

- Chopped fresh parsley for garnish (optional)

Instructions:

1. Heat olive oil in a pot over medium heat.

2. Sauté diced carrots, celery, and onions until softened. Add cooked lentils, vegetable broth, dried thyme, salt, and pepper to the pot.

3. Bring the mixture to a simmer and cook for 10-12 minutes. Adjust seasoning if needed.

4. Serve the lentil and vegetable soup hot, garnished with chopped fresh parsley if desired.

Shrimp and Avocado Salad

Ingredients:

• 4 oz cooked shrimp, peeled and deveined

• 1/2 avocado, sliced

• 2 cups mixed greens (such as spinach, arugula)

• 1/4 cup cherry tomatoes, halved

• 1 tablespoon olive oil

• 1 tablespoon lemon juice

• Salt and pepper to taste

Instructions:

1. In a bowl, combine mixed greens, cherry tomatoes, and cooked shrimp. Top with sliced avocado.

2. Drizzle olive oil and lemon juice over the salad. Season with salt and pepper according to taste.

3. Gently toss the salad until ingredients are well combined.

4. Serve this light and protein-rich shrimp and avocado salad.

Tofu Stir-Fry with Vegetables

Ingredients:

- 4 oz firm tofu, cubed

- 1/2 cup broccoli florets

- 1/2 cup sliced bell peppers (assorted colors)

- 1/4 cup sliced carrots

- 1/4 cup sliced mushrooms

- 2 tablespoons low-sodium soy sauce or tamari

- 1 tablespoon olive oil

- 1 teaspoon minced garlic

- 1/2 teaspoon grated ginger (optional)

Instructions:

1. Heat olive oil in a skillet or wok over medium-high heat.

2. Add minced garlic and grated ginger (if using), sautéing for a minute. Add cubed tofu to the skillet and cook until lightly browned.

3. Add broccoli florets, sliced bell peppers, carrots, and mushrooms to the skillet. Stir-fry for 4-5 minutes until the vegetables are tender yet crisp.

4. Pour low-sodium soy sauce or tamari over the stir-fry and toss to combine.

5. Serve this nutritious tofu and vegetable stir-fry immediately.

Tuna and Avocado Lettuce Wraps

Ingredients:

• 1 can (5 oz) tuna in water, drained

• 1/2 avocado, mashed

• 2 tablespoons diced red onions

• 2 tablespoons diced celery

• 1 tablespoon chopped fresh parsley

• 1 tablespoon lemon juice

• Salt and pepper to taste

• 4 large lettuce leaves (such as butter lettuce or iceberg)

Instructions:

1. In a bowl, combine drained tuna, mashed avocado, diced red onions, diced celery, chopped parsley, lemon juice, salt, and pepper. Mix well.

2. Lay out the lettuce leaves on a clean surface. Spoon the tuna and avocado mixture onto each lettuce leaf.

3. Wrap the lettuce leaves around the filling to create wraps. Secure with toothpicks if needed.

4. Serve these protein-packed and flavorful tuna and avocado lettuce wraps.

Chicken and Veggie Lettuce Cups

Ingredients:

• 4 oz cooked chicken breast, diced

• 1/4 cup diced bell peppers (assorted colors)

• 1/4 cup diced cucumbers

• 1/4 cup grated carrots

• 2 tablespoons sliced green onions

• 2 tablespoons low-fat Greek yogurt

• 1 tablespoon lime juice

- 1 teaspoon honey

- Salt and pepper to taste

- 4 large lettuce leaves (such as Bibb or Boston lettuce)

Instructions:

1. In a bowl, mix diced chicken breast, diced bell peppers, diced cucumbers, grated carrots, and sliced green onions.

2. In a separate small bowl, whisk together low-fat Greek yogurt, lime juice, honey, salt, and pepper.

3. Pour the dressing over the chicken and veggie mixture. Toss until well coated.

4. Lay out the lettuce leaves on a clean surface. Spoon the chicken and veggie mixture onto each lettuce leaf.

5. Fold the lettuce leaves around the filling to form cups.

6. Serve these refreshing and protein-rich chicken and veggie lettuce cups.

Turkey and Quinoa Stuffed Bell Peppers

Ingredients:

- 2 large bell peppers (any color), halved and seeds removed

- 1/2 cup cooked quinoa

- 4 oz cooked ground turkey

- 1/4 cup diced tomatoes

- 2 tablespoons diced onions

- 2 tablespoons shredded cheese (optional)

- 1 teaspoon olive oil

- Salt and pepper to taste

Instructions:

1. Preheat the oven to 375°F (190°C). Place the halved bell peppers in a baking dish.

2. In a skillet, heat olive oil over medium heat. Sauté diced tomatoes and onions until softened.

3. Add cooked ground turkey and cooked quinoa to the skillet. Season with salt and pepper. Cook until heated through.

4. Fill each bell pepper half with the turkey and quinoa mixture.

5. If desired, sprinkle shredded cheese on top of each stuffed pepper. Bake for 25-30 minutes or until the peppers are tender.

6. Serve these colorful and nutritious turkey and quinoa stuffed bell peppers.

Eggplant and Chickpea Salad

Ingredients:

- 1 medium eggplant, diced

- 1 can (15 oz) chickpeas, drained and rinsed

- 2 tablespoons olive oil

- 1 teaspoon smoked paprika

- 1/2 teaspoon garlic powder

- Salt and pepper to taste

- 2 cups mixed greens

- 2 tablespoons chopped fresh cilantro or parsley

- Lemon wedges for serving (optional)

Instructions:

1. Preheat the oven to 400°F (200°C). Line a baking sheet with parchment paper.

2. In a bowl, toss diced eggplant and chickpeas with olive oil, smoked paprika, garlic powder, salt, and pepper.

3. Spread the seasoned eggplant and chickpeas onto the prepared baking sheet in a single layer.

4. Roast in the oven for 25-30 minutes or until the eggplant is tender and slightly browned.

5. In a large bowl, mix the roasted eggplant and chickpeas with mixed greens and chopped cilantro or parsley.

6. Serve this flavorful eggplant and chickpea salad with lemon wedges if desired.

Ingredients:

- 4 oz firm tofu, cubed

- 1 cup broccoli florets

- 1/2 cup sliced bell peppers (assorted colors)

- 1/4 cup sliced carrots

- 1/4 cup sliced mushrooms

- 2 tablespoons low-sodium soy sauce or tamari

- 1 tablespoon olive oil

- 1 teaspoon minced garlic

- 1/2 teaspoon grated ginger (optional)

- Cooked brown rice or quinoa for serving (optional)

Instructions:

1. Heat olive oil in a skillet or wok over medium-high heat.

2. Add minced garlic and grated ginger (if using), sautéing for a minute. Add cubed tofu to the skillet and cook until lightly browned.

3. Add broccoli florets, sliced bell peppers, carrots, and mushrooms to the skillet. Stir-fry for 4-5 minutes until the vegetables are tender yet crisp.

4. Pour low-sodium soy sauce or tamari over the stir-fry and toss to combine.

5. Serve this nutritious veggie and tofu stir-fry as is or over cooked brown rice or quinoa.

Zucchini Noodles with Turkey Bolognese

Ingredients:

• 1 medium zucchini, spiralized into noodles

• 4 oz lean ground turkey

• 1/2 cup low-sodium marinara sauce

• 1 tablespoon olive oil

• 1 teaspoon minced garlic

• 1/2 teaspoon Italian seasoning

• Salt and pepper to taste

• Fresh basil leaves for garnish (optional)

Instructions:

1. Heat olive oil in a skillet over medium heat. Add minced garlic and cook for a minute.

2. Add ground turkey to the skillet, breaking it apart with a spatula, and cook until browned.

3. Stir in marinara sauce, Italian seasoning, salt, and pepper. Simmer for 5-7 minutes.

4. In a separate skillet, lightly sauté zucchini noodles until just tender. Plate the zucchini noodles and top with turkey Bolognese sauce.

5. Garnish with fresh basil leaves if desired. Enjoy this low-carb twist on spaghetti!

Shredded Chicken Lettuce Wraps

Ingredients:

• 4 oz cooked shredded chicken breast

• 1/4 cup diced tomatoes

• 2 tablespoons diced red onions

• 2 tablespoons diced bell peppers

• 2 tablespoons chopped cilantro

• 1 tablespoon lime juice

• Salt and pepper to taste

• 4 large lettuce leaves (such as butter lettuce)

Instructions:

1. In a bowl, mix shredded chicken, diced tomatoes, red onions, bell peppers, chopped cilantro, lime juice, salt, and pepper.

2. Lay out the lettuce leaves on a clean surface. Spoon the chicken mixture onto each lettuce leaf.

3. Wrap the lettuce leaves around the filling to create wraps.

4. Serve these refreshing and protein-packed chicken lettuce wraps.

Spinach and Feta Stuffed Portobello Mushrooms

Ingredients:

• 2 large portobello mushrooms, stems removed

• 1 cup fresh spinach, chopped

• 2 tablespoons diced onions

• 2 tablespoons crumbled feta cheese

• 1 tablespoon olive oil

• 1 teaspoon minced garlic

• Salt and pepper to taste

Instructions:

1. Preheat the oven to 375°F (190°C). Place the portobello mushrooms on a baking sheet, gill-side up.

2. In a skillet, heat olive oil over medium heat. Add minced garlic and diced onions, sautéing until softened.

3. Add chopped spinach to the skillet and cook until wilted. Season with salt and pepper.

4. Divide the spinach mixture evenly between the portobello mushroom caps. Top each mushroom with crumbled feta cheese.

5. Bake for 15-20 minutes or until the mushrooms are tender.

6. Serve these flavorful spinach and feta stuffed portobello mushrooms.

Turkey and Veggie Lettuce Wraps

Ingredients:

- 4 oz cooked ground turkey

- 1/4 cup diced bell peppers (assorted colors)

- 1/4 cup diced zucchini

- 1/4 cup diced tomatoes

- 2 tablespoons diced red onions

- 2 tablespoons low-sodium soy sauce or tamari

- 1 tablespoon olive oil

- 1 teaspoon minced garlic

- Salt and pepper to taste

- 4 large lettuce leaves (such as romaine or iceberg)

Instructions:

1. Heat olive oil in a skillet over medium heat. Add minced garlic and cook for a minute.

2. Add diced bell peppers, zucchini, tomatoes, and red onions to the skillet. Sauté until vegetables are tender.

3. Stir in cooked ground turkey, low-sodium soy sauce or tamari, salt, and pepper. Cook for another 2-3 minutes.

4. Lay out the lettuce leaves on a clean surface. Spoon the turkey and veggie mixture onto each lettuce leaf.

5. Wrap the lettuce leaves around the filling to create wraps.

6. Serve these delicious and protein-rich turkey and veggie lettuce wraps.

Tofu and Broccoli Stir-Fry

Ingredients:

- 4 oz firm tofu, cut into cubes

- 1 cup broccoli florets

- 1/4 cup sliced bell peppers (assorted colors)

- 2 tablespoons low-sodium soy sauce or tamari

- 1 tablespoon olive oil

- 1 teaspoon minced garlic

- 1/2 teaspoon grated ginger (optional)

- Cooked brown rice for serving (optional)

Instructions:

1. Heat olive oil in a skillet or wok over medium-high heat.

2. Add minced garlic and grated ginger (if using), sautéing for a minute. Add cubed tofu to the skillet and cook until lightly browned.

3. Add broccoli florets and sliced bell peppers to the skillet. Stir-fry for 4-5 minutes until vegetables are tender yet crisp.

4. Pour low-sodium soy sauce or tamari over the stir-fry and toss to combine.

5. Serve this nutritious tofu and broccoli stir-fry as is or over cooked brown rice.

Cauliflower Fried Rice

Ingredients:

- 1 cup cauliflower rice (fresh or frozen)

- 4 oz cooked chicken breast, diced

- 1/4 cup diced carrots

- 1/4 cup peas (fresh or frozen)

- 2 tablespoons diced onions

- 1 tablespoon low-sodium soy sauce or tamari

- 1 teaspoon sesame oil

- 1 teaspoon minced garlic

- 1 egg, beaten (optional)

- Salt and pepper to taste

- Chopped green onions for garnish (optional)

Instructions:

1. In a skillet, heat sesame oil over medium heat. Add minced garlic and diced onions, sautéing until fragrant.

2. Add diced carrots and peas to the skillet, cooking until slightly tender.

3. Push the veggies to one side of the skillet and pour the beaten egg (if using) onto the other side. Scramble the egg until cooked.

4. Add cooked chicken breast and cauliflower rice to the skillet. Stir-fry for 3-4 minutes.

5. Pour low-sodium soy sauce or tamari over the mixture. Toss until well combined.

6. Season with salt and pepper according to taste.

7. Garnish with chopped green onions if desired. Enjoy this low-carb cauliflower fried "rice".

Tofu and Vegetable Buddha Bowl

Ingredients:

• 4 oz firm tofu, sliced into cubes

• 1/2 cup cooked quinoa

• 1 cup mixed greens (such as kale, spinach)

• 1/4 cup shredded carrots

• 1/4 cup sliced cucumbers

• 2 tablespoons hummus or tahini (as a dressing)

• 1 tablespoon olive oil

• 1 tablespoon lemon juice

• Salt and pepper to taste

• Sesame seeds for garnish (optional)

Instructions:

1. In a skillet, heat olive oil over medium heat. Add tofu cubes and cook until lightly browned.

2. In a bowl, assemble mixed greens, cooked quinoa, shredded carrots, and sliced cucumbers.

3. Top the bowl with the cooked tofu cubes. Drizzle hummus or tahini, olive oil, and lemon juice over the ingredients.

4. Season with salt and pepper according to taste.

5. Garnish with sesame seeds if desired. Enjoy this vibrant and nutritious Buddha bowl.

Turkey and Black Bean Lettuce Cups

Ingredients:

• 4 oz cooked ground turkey

• 1/2 cup canned black beans, drained and rinsed

• 2 tablespoons diced tomatoes

• 2 tablespoons diced red onions

• 2 tablespoons chopped cilantro

- 1 tablespoon lime juice

- Salt and pepper to taste

- 4 large lettuce leaves (such as romaine or iceberg)

Instructions:

1. In a bowl, combine cooked ground turkey, black beans, diced tomatoes, red onions, chopped cilantro, lime juice, salt, and pepper.

2. Lay out the lettuce leaves on a clean surface. Spoon the turkey and black bean mixture onto each lettuce leaf.

3. Wrap the lettuce leaves around the filling to create cups.

4. Serve these protein-packed turkey and black bean lettuce cups.

Quinoa and Veggie Stir-Fry

Ingredients:

- 1/2 cup cooked quinoa

- 1 cup mixed vegetables (broccoli florets, bell peppers, snap peas)

- 2 tablespoons low-sodium soy sauce or tamari

- 1 tablespoon olive oil

- 1 teaspoon minced garlic

• 1/2 teaspoon grated ginger (optional)

• Sesame seeds for garnish (optional)

Instructions:

1. Heat olive oil in a skillet or wok over medium-high heat.

2. Add minced garlic and grated ginger (if using), sautéing for a minute. Add mixed vegetables to the skillet and stir-fry for 4-5 minutes until tender yet crisp.

3. Add cooked quinoa to the skillet and toss to combine with the vegetables. Pour low-sodium soy sauce or tamari over the mixture. Toss until well coated.

4. Garnish with sesame seeds if desired. Serve this flavorful quinoa and veggie stir-fry.

Caprese Stuffed Chicken Breast

Ingredients:

• 2 boneless, skinless chicken breasts

• 1/4 cup sliced cherry tomatoes

• 2 tablespoons shredded mozzarella cheese

• 2 tablespoons chopped fresh basil

• 1 tablespoon olive oil

• Salt and pepper to taste

Instructions:

1. Preheat the oven to 375°F (190°C).

2. Cut a pocket into each chicken breast without cutting all the way through.

3. Stuff each chicken breast with sliced cherry tomatoes, shredded mozzarella cheese, and chopped fresh basil.

4. Drizzle olive oil over the chicken breasts and season with salt and pepper.

5. Place the chicken breasts on a baking dish and bake for 25-30 minutes or until cooked through.

6. Serve these delicious caprese stuffed chicken breasts.

Turkey and Vegetable Skewers

Ingredients:

• 4 oz cooked turkey breast, cubed

• 1/2 cup cherry tomatoes

• 1/2 cup bell pepper chunks (assorted colors)

• 1/2 cup zucchini chunks

• 1 tablespoon olive oil

• 1 teaspoon minced garlic

• Salt and pepper to taste

• Wooden skewers

Instructions:

1. Preheat a grill or grill pan over medium-high heat.

2. Thread turkey cubes, cherry tomatoes, bell pepper chunks, and zucchini chunks onto wooden skewers in alternating patterns.

3. In a small bowl, mix olive oil, minced garlic, salt, and pepper. Brush the skewers with the olive oil mixture.

4. Grill the skewers for 8-10 minutes, turning occasionally, until the turkey is heated through and the vegetables are slightly charred.

5. Serve these flavorful turkey and vegetable skewers.

Spinach and Feta Stuffed Chicken Breast

Ingredients:

• 2 boneless, skinless chicken breasts

• 1 cup fresh spinach leaves

• 2 tablespoons crumbled feta cheese

• 1 tablespoon olive oil

• 1 teaspoon minced garlic

• Salt and pepper to taste

Instructions:

1. Preheat the oven to 375°F (190°C).

2. In a skillet, heat olive oil over medium heat. Add minced garlic and cook for a minute.

3. Add fresh spinach leaves to the skillet and cook until wilted. Season with salt and pepper.

4. Cut a pocket into each chicken breast without cutting all the way through. Stuff each chicken breast with the cooked spinach and crumbled feta cheese.

5. Season the outside of the chicken breasts with salt and pepper.

6. Place the chicken breasts on a baking dish and bake for 25-30 minutes or until cooked through.

7. Serve these delicious spinach and feta stuffed chicken breasts.

Tuna Salad Lettuce Wraps

Ingredients:

• 1 can (5 oz) tuna in water, drained

• 2 tablespoons diced celery

• 2 tablespoons diced red onions

• 2 tablespoons chopped pickles

• 2 tablespoons low-fat Greek yogurt

• 1 tablespoon lemon juice

• Salt and pepper to taste

• 4 large lettuce leaves (such as Bibb or Boston lettuce)

Instructions:

1. In a bowl, mix drained tuna, diced celery, diced red onions, chopped pickles, low-fat Greek yogurt, lemon juice, salt, and pepper.

2. Lay out the lettuce leaves on a clean surface. Spoon the tuna salad mixture onto each lettuce leaf.

3. Wrap the lettuce leaves around the filling to create wraps.

4. Serve these refreshing and protein-rich tuna salad lettuce wraps.

Veggie and Quinoa Stuffed Bell Peppers

Ingredients:

• 2 large bell peppers (any color), halved and seeds removed

• 1 cup cooked quinoa

• 1/2 cup black beans, drained and rinsed

- 1/4 cup diced tomatoes

- 2 tablespoons diced onions

- 2 tablespoons shredded cheese (optional)

- 1 tablespoon olive oil

- Salt and pepper to taste

Instructions:

1. Preheat the oven to 375°F (190°C). Place the halved bell peppers in a baking dish.

2. In a skillet, heat olive oil over medium heat. Sauté diced tomatoes and onions until softened.

3. Add cooked quinoa, black beans, and optional shredded cheese to the skillet. Season with salt and pepper. Cook until heated through.

4. Fill each bell pepper half with the quinoa and veggie mixture.

5. If desired, sprinkle shredded cheese on top of each stuffed pepper. Bake for 25-30 minutes or until the peppers are tender.

6. Serve these colorful and nutritious veggie and quinoa stuffed bell peppers.

Egg Drop Soup

Ingredients:

• 4 cups low-sodium chicken or vegetable broth

• 2 large eggs, beaten

• 1/4 cup diced green onions

• 1 teaspoon low-sodium soy sauce or tamari

• 1/2 teaspoon grated ginger (optional)

• Salt and pepper to taste

Instructions:

1. In a pot, bring the chicken or vegetable broth to a gentle simmer over medium heat.

2. While stirring the broth, slowly pour in the beaten eggs in a thin stream to create egg ribbons.

3. Add diced green onions, low-sodium soy sauce or tamari, grated ginger (if using), salt, and pepper.

4. Cook for an additional 2-3 minutes until the soup is heated through.

5. Serve this comforting and protein-rich egg drop soup.

Skillet Salsa Shrimp With Spinach and Feta

Ingredients:

- 1 tbsp. olive oil

- 4 cloves garlic, finely chopped

- 3 strips lemon zest, thinly sliced

- 1/2 15.5 oz. jar salsa

- 8 oz. tomato sauce

- 20 shrimp, peeled and deveined

- 2 c. baby spinach

- 1/4 c. crumbled feta, for serving

- flatbread, for serving

Instructions:

1. Heat olive oil, garlic, and lemon zest in a large skillet on medium until beginning to brown, about 1 min.

2. Add salsa and tomato sauce and bring to a simmer. Nestle shrimp in the salsa mixture and cook, covered, 3 min.

3. Fold in spinach and cook until beginning to wilt and shrimp are opaque throughout, 1 to 2 min. more.

4. Sprinkle with feta and serve with flatbread if desired.

Ingredients:

- 2 tbsp. olive oil

- 4 cloves garlic, finely chopped

- 2 tsp. vegetable bouillon base (we used Better Than Bouillon)

- 12 oz. orecchiette pasta

- 2 tsp. fresh thyme leaves

- 1 14-oz. can small white beans, rinsed

- 2 c. baby spinach

- 1/2 c. finely grated Parmesan cheese

- pepper

Instructions:

1. Heat oil and garlic in large deep skillet on medium until garlic is light golden brown, about 2 min. Remove from heat, add 4 cups water, and whisk in bouillon base.

2. Add orecchiette and thyme and bring to a boil. Reduce heat and simmer, stirring frequently, until orecchiette is al dente, 10 to 12 min.

3. Fold in beans, spinach, Parmesan, and 1/2 tsp. pepper and cook until beans are heated through, about 2 min.

Ingredients:

- 1 lb. boneless, skinless chicken breasts, cut into thin strips

- 1 tsp. ground cumin

- 1 tsp. chili powder

- kosher salt

- pepper

- 1 tbsp. canola oil

- 1 red pepper, sliced

- 1 small onion, sliced

- 1 c. sliced mushrooms

- 3 cloves garlic, chopped

- 1 tbsp. chopped chipotle chiles in adobo

Chiles in adobo

- 1 1/2 tbsp. fresh lime juice

- 8 flour tortillas, warmed

- grated cheddar cheese, for serving

- cilantro, for serving

- lime wedges, for serving

Instructions:

1. Season chicken with cumin, chili powder, and 1/4 tsp. each salt and pepper. Heat oil in large cast-iron skillet on medium-high. Add chicken and cook, stirring occasionally, until cooked through, 5 to 7 min. Transfer to plate.

2. To same skillet, add red pepper, onion, mushrooms, and garlic and cook, stirring occasionally, until soft, 4 to 6 min. Stir in chipotle chiles, lime juice, chicken, and a pinch each of salt and pepper. Cook, stirring, until heated through.

3. Serve chicken and vegetables with tortillas and toppings.

Roasted Chicken and Potatoes With Kale

Ingredients:

- 1 lb. yellow potatoes, cut into 3/4-in. pieces

- 1/2 c. green olives

- 2 tsp. fresh thyme leaves

- 3 tbsp. olive oil, divided

- kosher salt

- pepper

- 1 lemon, halved

- 1 tsp. paprika

- 4 small chicken legs, split (4 drumsticks and 4 thighs; about 2 1/2 lbs.)

- 4 c. baby kale

Instructions:

1. Heat oven to 425°F. On large rimmed baking sheet, toss potatoes, olives, and thyme with 2 tbsp. oil and 1/4 tsp. each salt and pepper. Place lemon halves, cut sides down, on baking sheet.

2. In small bowl, combine paprika, remaining tbsp. oil, and 1/2 tsp. each salt and pepper. Rub mixture all over chicken and transfer chicken to baking sheet, nestling among vegetables.

3. Roast chicken and vegetables until chicken is golden brown and cooked through, 25 to 30 min.

4. Transfer chicken to plates, scatter kale over vegetables in pan, and return to oven until kale is just beginning to wilt, about 1 min. Fold kale into potatoes, squeeze juice of lemon over vegetables, and serve with chicken.

Veggies on Sweet Potato Mash

Ingredients:

- 2 lb. sweet potatoes (about 4 large), peeled and cut into 1-in. chunks

- Kosher salt and pepper

- 3 oz. Greek yogurt

- 2 tbsp. unsalted butter

- 1 tbsp. olive oil

- 12 oz. mini sweet peppers, sliced

- 3 cloves garlic, chopped

- 1 bunch curly kale (about 11 oz.), ribs removed, leaves chopped

- 1 15-oz. can pinto beans, rinsed

- 1 tbsp. fresh lemon juice

- 1 tbsp. Worcestershire sauce

- 1/4 c. roasted sunflower seeds

Instructions:

1. Place potatoes in large pot, cover with cold water, and bring to a boil. Add 2 tsp salt, reduce heat, and simmer until tender, 10 to 12 min. Drain potatoes and return to pot; mash with yogurt and butter.

2. Meanwhile, heat oil in Dutch oven or second large pot on medium. Stir in peppers and garlic, then add kale and 1/2 tsp. salt and cook, tossing and stirring often, until kale is just wilted, 8 to 10 min.

3. Add beans, lemon juice, Worcestershire sauce, and 1/2 tsp pepper and cook until beans are just heated through., about 2 min. Serve over mash and sprinkle with sunflower seeds.

Fish Chowder Sheet Pan Bake

Ingredients:

- 1 lb. small yellow potatoes (about 16), halved lengthwise

- 2 small red onions, cut into 1/2-in.-thick wedges

- 4 slices bacon, cut into 1/2-in. pieces

- 1 tbsp. mayonnaise

- 1 tbsp. Dijon mustard

- 1 tsp. finely grated lemon zest

- 1/4 c. panko

- 1 tbsp. olive oil

- 1 tbsp. fresh thyme leaves

- 4 6-oz. pieces cod fillet (at least 1 in. thick)

- pepper

Instructions:

1. Heat oven to 450°F. Pile potatoes and onions in center of rimmed baking sheet and place bacon on top. Roast 10 min.

2. Meanwhile, in small bowl, combine mayonnaise, mustard, and lemon zest. In second bowl, combine panko with oil, then fold in thyme. Season fish with 1/2 tsp pepper; spread with mayo mixture and sprinkle with panko.

3. Remove baking sheet from oven and reduce oven temp to 425°F. Toss potatoes, onions, and bacon together, then spread in even layer, arranging potatoes cut sides down.

4. Nestle fish pieces among vegetables and roast until fish is opaque throughout and potatoes are golden brown and tender, 12 to 15 min.

Seared Tilapia With Spiralized Zucchini

Ingredients:

• 1 1/2 lb. zucchini

• 3 tbsp. olive oil, divided

• kosher salt

• pepper

• 4 small fillets tilapia (1 1/2 lbs.)

• 1 lemon, thinly sliced and seeded

• 2 cloves garlic, thinly sliced

• 1 tbsp. capers

• 1/2 c. fresh flat-leaf parsley, chopped

Instructions:

1. Heat oven to 475°F. Line large rimmed baking sheet with reusable baking mat or parchment paper. Using spiralizer, spiralize zucchini, or slice zucchini into thin ribbons.

2. Transfer zucchini to prepared baking sheet; toss with 1 tbsp. oil and 1/4 tsp. each salt and pepper. Roast 15 min. Increase heat to broil and continue to cook until golden brown, 3 to 4 min.

3. Meanwhile, heat 1 tbsp. oil in large cast-iron skillet on medium-high. Season fish with 1/4 tsp. each salt and pepper and cook until just opaque throughout, 2 to 3 min. per side. Transfer to plates.

4. Add remaining tbsp. oil to skillet along with lemon, garlic, and capers and cook, stirring occasionally, until garlic is golden brown and tender. Toss with parsley, then spoon over tilapia and serve with zucchini.

Striped Bass With Radish Salsa Verde

Ingredients:

• 1 small clove garlic, pressed

• 1 tbsp. anchovy paste (or 3 anchovy fillets, finely chopped)

• 1/2 small red onion, finely chopped

• 1 tbsp. red wine vinegar

• 1/2 c. plus 1 tbsp. olive oil, divided

- 1 bunch radishes, diced, leaves separated and finely chopped

- 1 c. flat-leaf parsley leaves, finely chopped

- 1 tsp. tarragon leaves, finely chopped

- 4 6-oz. fillets striped bass

- kosher salt

- pepper

Instructions:

1. In medium bowl, whisk together garlic, anchovy paste, onion, and vinegar and let sit 5 min.

2. Stir in 1/2 cup oil, then radishes, radish greens, parsley, and tarragon.

3. Heat remaining tbsp. oil in medium skillet on medium. Pat fish dry and season with 1/2 tsp. each salt and pepper. Cook, skin side down, until skin is crisp and golden brown, about 6 min. Flip and cook until fish is just opaque throughout, 2 to 4 min. more. Serve topped with radish salsa verde.

Greek Salad Pasta

Ingredients:

- 1/2 lb. orecchiette

- 4 thin sliced chicken cutlets (about 12 ounces total)

- Kosher salt and ground black pepper

- 3 tbsp. extra-virgin olive oil

- 2 tbsp. red wine vinegar

- 1 tsp. dried oregano

- Kosher salt and ground black pepper

- 1/2 English cucumber, cut into half moons

- 1 c. halved cherry tomatoes

- 1/2 c. pitted kalamata olives

- 1/2 small red onion, thinly sliced

- 1/4 c. crumbled feta cheese

- 1 tbsp. chopped fresh dill

Instructions:

1. Bring a pot of well-salted water to a boil. Cook the pasta according to package directions. Season the chicken with salt and pepper. Heat a grill pan over medium high and spray the grill pan with cooking spray.

2. Add the chicken and cook until good grill marks form, about 5 minutes. Flip and continue to cook until cooked through, about 4 minutes more. Transfer the chicken to a cutting board and cut into bite size pieces.

3. In a large bowl, whisk together the olive oil, vinegar, oregano, a pinch of salt, and a few grinds of pepper. Add the cucumber, tomatoes, olives, onion, feta, and dill.

4. Drain the pasta and toss into the vegetables in the bowl with the chicken to combine. Season to taste with salt and pepper and serve hot, cold, or room temperature.

Seared Salmon with Roasted Cauliflower

Ingredients:

Cauliflower

• 1 large head cauliflower

• 2 tbsp. olive oil

• 1/4 tsp. salt

• 1/4 tsp. pepper

Salmon

• 4 six-oz. pieces salmon

• 2 tsp. olive oil

• 2 cloves garlic, chopped

• 1 tbsp. capers

• 1/2 c. parsley leaves

Instructions:

1. Toss cauliflower florets with olive oil, salt, and pepper.

2. Roast at 450°F until tender, then broil until golden brown.

3. Season and cook salmon in oil in a large skillet on medium-high, until opaque throughout, adding garlic and capers to the skillet after flipping salmon once.

4. Toss cauliflower with capers, garlic, and parsley leaves; serve with salmon.

Shrimp, Avocado, and Egg Chopped Salad

Ingredients:

- 1/4 small red onion, thinly sliced

- 2 tbsp. fresh lime juice

- 1 tbsp. olive oil

- 12 oz. large peeled and deveined shrimp

- Kosher salt and pepper

- 1 c. grape tomatoes, halved

- 8 c. butter lettuce

- 1/2 c. fresh cilantro leaves

- 1/2 avocado, diced

• 2 hard boiled eggs, cut into pieces

Instructions:

1. In a large bowl, toss onion with lime juice and ½ tablespoon oil and let sit for 5 minutes.

2. Heat 1/2 tablespoon oil in a large skillet on medium high. Season shrimp with 1/4 teaspoon each salt and pepper and cook until opaque throughout, 2 to 3 minutes per side.

3. Toss tomatoes with onions, then toss with lettuce and cilantro. Divide among bowls and top with shrimp, avocado and egg.

Spiced Grilled Eggplant with Fresh Tomato Salad

Ingredients:

• 2 medium eggplants (about 1 lb each), sliced lengthwise 1/2 inch thick

• 4 tbsp. olive oil

• 1 tsp. ground coriander

• 1 tsp. cayenne Kosher salt

• 2 tbsp. fresh lemon juice

• 2 tbsp. red wine vinegar

• 1 1/2 c. multicolored cherry or grape tomatoes, halved

- 2 small Fresno chiles or other hot chiles, finely chopped

- 1/4 c. packed fresh mint leaves, finely chopped, plus more for serving

- 1/4 c. low-fat Greek yogurt

- 2 tbsp. low-fat milk

Instructions:

1. Heat grill to medium. Brush eggplant with 3 Tbsp oil, then season with coriander, cayenne, and 1/4 tsp salt. Grill until tender, 10 to 12 minutes.

2. Meanwhile, in a medium bowl, whisk together lemon juice, vinegar, remaining Tbsp oil, and 1/2 tsp salt; fold in tomatoes, chiles, and mint.

3. Arrange eggplant on a large platter; top with tomato salad. Whisk together yogurt and milk and drizzle over vegetables. Sprinkle with mint leaves if desired.

Seared Tilapia With Spiralized Zucchini

Ingredients:

- 1 1/2 lb. zucchini

- 3 tbsp. olive oil, divided

- kosher salt

- pepper

- 4 small fillets tilapia (1 1/2 lbs.)

- 1 lemon, thinly sliced and seeded

- 2 cloves garlic, thinly sliced

- 1 tbsp. capers

- 1/2 c. fresh flat-leaf parsley, chopped

Instructions:

1. Heat oven to 475°F. Line large rimmed baking sheet with reusable baking mat or parchment paper. Using spiralizer, spiralize zucchini, or slice zucchini into thin ribbons.

2. Transfer zucchini to prepared baking sheet; toss with 1 tbsp. oil and 1/4 tsp. each salt and pepper. Roast 15 min. Increase heat to broil and continue to cook until golden brown, 3 to 4 min.

3. Meanwhile, heat 1 tbsp. oil in large cast-iron skillet on medium-high. Season fish with 1/4 tsp. each salt and pepper and cook until just opaque throughout, 2 to 3 min. per side. Transfer to plates.

4. Add remaining tbsp. oil to skillet along with lemon, garlic, and capers and cook, stirring occasionally, until garlic is golden brown and tender. Toss with parsley, then spoon over tilapia and serve with zucchini.

Pan-Roasted Bass With Papaya Relish

Ingredients:

* 2 scallions

* 2 tbsp. plus 1 tsp olive oil

* 1 tbsp. lime juice

* 1 tsp. honey

* Kosher salt

* 1 jalapeño, thinly sliced

* 4 6-oz fillets striped bass

* 1 c. diced papaya (about 1 small papaya)

* 1 avocado, diced

Instructions:

1. Heat broiler. Place scallions on a rimmed baking sheet, drizzle with 1 tsp oil, and broil until charred, about 2 minutes. Transfer to a cutting board, let cool, then thinly slice.

2. In a large bowl, whisk together lime juice, honey, and 1/4 tsp salt. Stir in jalapeño and scallions.

3. Heat remaining 2Tbsp oil in a medium skillet on medium. Pat fish dry, season with 1/2 tsp each salt and pepper, and cook, skin side down, until skin is golden brown and crisp, 6 to 7 minutes. Flip and cook until fish is opaque throughout, 3 to 5 minutes more. Transfer to a platter.

4. Fold papaya and avocado into jalapeño mixture and spoon over fish.

Roasted Sweet Potato and Chicken Salad

Ingredients:

- 2 1/2 lb. sweet potatoes, cut into 1/2-inch chunks

- 2 tbsp. olive oil

- 1/4 tsp. salt

- 1/4 c. seasoned rice vinegar

- 2 tbsp. toasted sesame oil

- 1 tbsp. miso paste

- 1 tbsp. finely chopped peeled fresh ginger

- 1/4 tsp. pepper

- 20 oz. mixed greens

- 2 rotisserie chicken-breast halves (about 8 oz.), sliced

- 1 avocado, sliced

- Sesame seeds, for garnish

Instructions:

1. On large rimmed baking sheet, toss sweet potatoes with olive oil and salt; roast in 450 degrees F oven 25 minutes or until tender.

2. Whisk together rice vinegar, sesame oil, miso, ginger and pepper.

3. Among four plates layered with 5 oz. mixed greens, divide sweet potatoes, rotisserie chicken and avocado. Drizzle with miso vinaigrette; top with sesame seeds.

Seared Coconut-Lime Chicken with Snap Pea Slaw

Ingredients:

- 2 tbsp. toasted sesame oil

- 1 tbsp. grated fresh ginger

- 3 tbsp. fresh lime juice, divided (from about 2 limes)

- Kosher salt and pepper

- 10 oz. snap peas, strings removed and thinly sliced

- 4 oz. snow peas, thinly sliced

- 2 scallions, thinly sliced

- 2 8-ounce boneless, skinless chicken breasts

- 1 tbsp. olive oil

- 2 tbsp. coconut cream

- 1/2 c. cilantro

Instructions:

1. In large bowl, whisk together sesame oil, ginger, 1 1/2 tablespoons lime juice and 1/2 teaspoon salt. Add snap peas, snow peas and scallions, and toss to combine.

2. Cut each breast horizontally in half to make 4 thin cutlets, then pound to 1/4 inch thick. Heat oil in large skillet on medium-high. Season chicken with 1/2 teaspoon each salt and pepper and cook in batches until golden brown and cooked through, about 2 minutes per side.

3. Transfer chicken to plates as it is cooked. Remove pan from heat and stir in coconut cream and remaining 11/2 tablespoons lime juice, scraping up any browned bits. Spoon over chicken on plates.

4. Fold cilantro into pea mixture and serve on top of chicken.

Fiery Black Bean Soup

Ingredients:

- 8 oz. tomatillos (about 4), halved

- 2 cloves garlic, unpeeled

- 1 large yellow onion, cut into 1-in.-thick wedges

- 1 large poblano pepper, halved and seeded

* 1 jalapeño, halved and seeded

* 1 tbsp. olive oil

* kosher salt

* pepper

* 1/2 tsp. ground cumin

* 1/2 tsp. ground coriander

* 4 c. low-sodium chicken broth

* 2 15-oz. cans low-sodium black beans, rinsed

* 1 14.5-oz. can fire-roasted diced tomatoes, drained

* 1 small red onion, thinly sliced

* 2 tbsp. fresh lime juice

* cilantro leaves, for serving

Instructions:

1. Heat broiler. On large rimmed baking sheet, toss tomatillos, garlic, yellow onion, poblano, and jalapeño with oil and 1/2 tsp. each salt and pepper. Turn peppers cut sides down and broil, rotating pan every 5 min., until vegetables are tender and charred, 15 min.

2. Discard skins from poblanos and garlic. Finely chop vegetables and transfer to Dutch oven. Add cumin and coriander and cook on medium, stirring occasionally, 2 min.

Add broth, beans, and tomatoes and bring to a simmer; cook 4 min.

3. Meanwhile, toss red onion with lime juice and a pinch each of salt and pepper; let sit at least 10 min. Serve soup topped with pickled onions and cilantro.

White Wine and Tomato Mussels

Ingredients:

• 2 tbsp. olive oil

• 2 large cloves garlic, finely chopped

• 1 red chile, finely chopped

• 1 c. dry white wine

• 1/4 tsp. kosher salt

• 2 lb. mussels, scrubbed and beards removed

• 2 medium tomatoes (about 1 lb. total), seeded and chopped

• 1/2 c. basil, chopped

• 1/2 c. parsley, chopped

Instructions:

1. In large Dutch oven, heat olive oil, garlic, and red chile on medium-low, 3 min. Add white wine; boil 2 min.

2. Add kosher salt, then mussels, and cook, covered, stirring once or twice, until shells open, about 4 min. Transfer mussels to shallow bowl.

3. Add tomatoes and cook 2 min. Remove from heat and toss with basil and parsley, then spoon over mussels.

Roasted Cauliflower "Steak" Salad

Ingredients:

- 2 tbsp. olive oil, divided

- 2 tsp. za'atar spice blend

- 1 tsp. ground cumin

- Kosher salt

- pepper

- 2 large heads cauliflower (about 3 lbs. each), trimmed of outer leaves

- 2 large carrots

- 8 oz. dandelion greens, tough stems removed

- 1/2 c. plain, low-fat Greek yogurt

- 2 tbsp. tahini

- 2 tbsp. fresh lemon juice

• 1 clove garlic, minced

Instructions:

1. Heat oven to 450°F. Brush a large baking sheet with 1/2 Tbsp oil. In a small bowl, combine za'atar, cumin, and 1 tsp each salt and pepper.

2. Place 1 head cauliflower on a cutting board, stem side down. Cut down middle, through core and stem, then cut two 1-in.-thick "steaks" from middle. Repeat with other cauliflower head. Set aside remaining cauliflower for another use.

3. Brush both sides of steaks with remaining olive oil, season with spice mixture, and place on oiled baking sheet. Roast until bottom is deep golden brown, 25 to 30 minutes. Flip and bake until tender, 10 to 15 minutes more.

4. Meanwhile, using a vegetable peeler, peel carrots into ribbons and place in a large bowl along with dandelion greens.

5. In a small bowl, combine yogurt, tahini, lemon juice, garlic, 1 Tbsp water, 1/2 tsp salt, and 1/4 tsp pepper. Add 3 Tbsp of dressing to carrot mixture and, with hands or a spoon, massage dressing into greens and carrots for 5 minutes.

6. Place cauliflower steaks on plates, drizzle with remaining dressing, and top with salad.

Ingredients:

- 2 tbsp. extra-virgin olive oil

- 1 lb. shrimp, peeled and deveined

- Kosher salt

- Freshly ground black pepper

- 1 tbsp. sesame oil

- 1 small head broccoli, cut into small florets

- 8 oz. sugar snap peas

- 1 red bell pepper, sliced

- 3 cloves garlic, minced

- 1 tbsp. minced ginger

- 1/2 c. low-sodium soy sauce

- 1 tbsp. cornstarch

- Juice of 1 lime

- 2 tbsp. packed brown sugar

- Pinch red pepper flakes

Instructions:

1. In a large skillet over medium heat, heat olive oil. Add shrimp and season with salt and pepper. Cook until pink, 5 minutes, then remove from skillet.

2. Return skillet to heat and heat sesame oil. Add broccoli, peas, and bell pepper and cook until soft, 7 minutes. Add garlic and ginger and cook until fragrant, 1 minute more.

3. In a small bowl, whisk together soy sauce, cornstarch, lime juice, brown sugar, and a pinch of red pepper flakes. Add to skillet and toss to coat. Add shrimp and cook until heated through, 2 minutes.

Mediterranean Baked Cod

Ingredients:

• 1 tbsp. olive oil

• 1 medium onion, thinly sliced

• 6 oz. mini sweet peppers, halved lengthwise

• 1 pt. grape tomatoes, halved lengthwise

• 8 sprigs fresh thyme

• 1 1/2 lb. cod fillet

• 1/2 tsp. salt

• 1/2 tsp. pepper

Instructions:

1. Heat oven to 450°F. Heat oil in a large oven-safe skillet or Dutch oven on medium-high. Add onion, peppers, and 1/4 tsp each salt and pepper and cook, stirring occasionally, 5 minutes.

2. Add tomatoes and thyme and cook, tossing, 2 minutes; stir in 1/4 cup water and remove from heat.

3. Season cod with 1/4 tsp each salt and pepper and nestle among vegetables. Cover skillet, transfer to oven, and roast until cod is opaque throughout, 12 to 15 minutes.

Peach and Cucumber Salad

Ingredients:

• 2 tbsp. olive oil

• 1 tbsp. white wine vinegar

• 1/4 tsp. kosher salt

• 1/4 tsp. pepper

• 1 small shallot

• 1/2 small red chile

• 2 ripe peaches or nectarines

• 1 Kirby cucumber

• 1/4 c. basil

- 1/4 c. mint

Instructions:

1. In a bowl, whisk together olive oil, white wine vinegar, salt, and pepper.

2. Stir in shallot and red chile, both thinly sliced.

3. Cut peaches or nectarines into half-inch thick wedges and add them into the bowl. Let them sit and toss occasionally for five minutes.

4. Use a vegetable peeler to cut a Kirby cucumber into long, thin strips

5. Fold the cucumbers into peaches along with fresh basil and torn fresh mint.

Kale and Roasted Cauliflower Salad

Ingredients:

CAULIFLOWER TOPPING

- 1 lb. cauliflower florets

- 2 tbsp. extra virgin olive oil

SALAD

- 1/4 c. lemon juice

- 3 tbsp. extra virgin olive oil

- 1 bunch kale, ribs removed, chopped

- 1/4 small red onion, very thinly sliced

- 1/3 c. crumbled feta cheese

- 1/3 c. golden raisins

- 1/3 c. pine nuts

Instructions:

1. On a large rimmed baking sheet, toss cauliflower florets with olive oil and 1/8 teaspoon each of salt and pepper. Roast in 450°F oven for 25 minutes, or until stems are tender.

2. In large bowl, whisk lemon juice, olive oil and 1/2 teaspoon salt. Toss kale with dressing. Let stand at least 5 minutes.

3. To kale, add cooked cauliflower, onion, feta cheese, golden raisins and toasted pine nuts. Toss until well combined.

Ceviche-Style Passion Fruit Shrimp

Ingredients:

- 1/4 c. frozen passion fruit pulp, thawed

- 1 1/2 tbsp. fresh lime juice

- Kosher salt

- 1 large poblano pepper, chopped

- 1 small red onion, chopped

- 1/2 serrano chile, thinly sliced

- 1 lb. large peeled and deveined cooked shrimp

- 1 small avocado, diced

- 1/2 c. cilantro, roughly chopped

Instructions:

1. In a bowl, combine passion fruit pulp, lime juice, and ½ teaspoon salt. Mix in pepper, onion, and serrano chile.

2. Toss with shrimp, then avocado and cilantro. Refrigerate at least 10 minutes and up to 30 minutes before serving.

Shrimp Scampi with Zoodles

Ingredients:

- 6 oz. linguine

- 1 1/2 lb. peeled, deveined large shrimp

- 4 cloves garlic, grated

- 2 tbsp. olive oil

- Kosher salt and pepper

- 1 tbsp. lemon zest

- 2 tbsp. lemon juice (from 1 to 2 large lemons)

- 1/4 tsp. red pepper flakes

- 1/2 c. dry white wine

- 1 tbsp. unsalted butter

- 12 oz. zucchini (about 3), spiralized on the thickest setting

- 1/4 c. flat-leaf parsley, chopped

Instructions:

1. Cook pasta per pkg. directions. Reserve 1/4 cup cooking water, drain pasta, and return it to the pot.

2. Meanwhile, in a large bowl, toss shrimp, garlic, olive oil, 1/4 tsp salt, and 1/2 tsp pepper. Let sit at least 5 minutes.

3. Heat a large skillet on medium. Add shrimp mixture and cook until just barely opaque throughout, 3 to 4 minutes per side. Transfer to a plate, leaving any oil in the skillet.

4. Add lemon zest and pepper flakes and cook, stirring, 30 seconds. Add wine, scraping up any browned bits, then reduce by half. Stir in lemon juice and butter, then add zucchini noodles and simmer 2 minutes.

5. Return shrimp to the skillet along with pasta and toss to combine, adding some reserved pasta water if mixture seems dry. Sprinkle with parsley.

Ingredients:

- 1 lb. Italian eggplant, cut into 1-in. pieces

- Kosher salt and pepper

- 2 tbsp. olive oil, divided

- 1 bell pepper, cut into 1-in. pieces

- 4 cloves garlic, pressed

- 1 1/2 lb. sirloin steak, cut into 4 pieces

- 1/4 c. balsamic vinegar

- 1 small tomato

- 1/4 c. basil, thinly sliced

Instructions:

1. Heat oven to 400°F. Season eggplant all over with 1/2 tsp salt and let sit 5 minutes.

2. Heat 1/2 Tbsp oil in a large skillet on medium-high. In two batches, cook eggplant, tossing occasionally, until golden brown on all sides, 4 to 5 minutes. Transfer to a plate, reserving any oil left in the skillet. Add 1/2 Tbsp oil and repeat with remaining eggplant.

3. Add bell pepper and garlic to skillet, reduce heat to medium and cook, covered, stirring occasionally, until tender, 8 to 10

minutes, adding a splash of water to the skillet if they begin to stick.

4. Meanwhile, pat steaks dry. Heat remaining Tbsp oil in a large skillet on medium-high. Season steaks with 1/4 tsp each salt and pepper and cook until golden brown on all sides, 6 to 8 minutes total. Remove from heat and drain off any oil.

5. Add vinegar to skillet, then transfer to oven and cook, flipping steak once, to desired doneness, about 8 minutes for medium-rare. Transfer to a cutting board and let rest at least 5 minutes before slicing.

6. Return eggplant to the skillet with pepper mixture and cook, tossing occasionally, 2 minutes. Coarsely grate tomato directly into skillet and bring to a simmer. Fold in basil and serve with steak.

Oven-Roasted Salmon with Charred Lemon Vinaigrette

Ingredients:

• 1 lemon

• 2 bulbs fennel, thinly sliced

• 2 small red onions, thinly sliced

• 2 1/2 tbsp. olive oil, divided

• Kosher salt and pepper

• 1 1/4 lb. skin-on salmon fillet

- 1 tsp. stone-ground mustard

- 3 c. baby arugula

Instructions:

1. Heat broiler. Cut pointed ends off lemon, halve crosswise, and place on a rimmed baking sheet, center cut sides up. Broil on top rack until charred, 5 minutes; transfer to a plate and set aside.

2. Reduce oven temperature to 400°F. On rimmed baking sheet, toss fennel and onions with 1 1/2 Tbsp oil and 1/4 tsp each salt and pepper; arrange around edges of sheet.

3. Place salmon in center of sheet and season with 1/4 tsp each salt and pepper. Roast until vegetables are tender and salmon is opaque throughout, 17 to 20 minutes.

4. Juice charred lemon halves into a small bowl and whisk in mustard and remaining Tbsp oil. Remove baking sheet from oven and fold arugula into vegetables. Drizzle charred lemon vinaigrette over fish and vegetables and gently toss vegetables.

Skinny Alfredo

Ingredients

- 12 oz. whole-wheat linguine

- 1 tbsp. extra-virgin olive oil

- 3 cloves garlic, minced

- 2 tbsp. all-purpose flour

- 1 c. low-sodium chicken broth

- 3/4 c. 1% milk

- 1/2 c. freshly grated Parmesan

- 2 tbsp. plain Greek yogurt (optional)

- Freshly ground black pepper

- Pinch crushed red pepper flakes

- Freshly chopped parsley, for serving

Instructions:

1. In a large pot of salted boiling water, cook linguine according to package directions until al dente. Set aside ½ cup of pasta water, then drain pasta and set aside.

2. In a large skillet over medium heat, heat oil. Add garlic and cook until fragrant, 1 minute. Sprinkle flour over evenly, then stir and cook until mixture is lightly golden.

3. Very gradually add broth in while whisking, 2 tablespoons at a time, waiting for mixture to become completely smooth before adding more broth.

4. Bring mixture to a boil, then gradually stream in milk while whisking. Bring to a simmer and cook until sauce is thickened, 2 to 3 minutes.

5. Remove from heat and add Parmesan and yogurt, if using. Season with salt, pepper, and a pinch of red pepper flakes.

6. Add pasta and a 1/4 cup reserved pasta water to sauce and toss to combine. If sauce is too thick add more pasta water, a tablespoon at a time, until desired consistency.

7. Garnish with parsley before serving.

Cilantro Lime Salmon Bowls

Ingredients

- 3 red peppers, sliced into strips

- 2/3 c. olive oil, plus 1 tablespoon

- kosher salt

- Freshly ground black pepper

- 1/3 c. lime juice

- 2 tbsp. finely chopped cilantro, plus more for serving

- 2 tsp. honey

- 1 Garlic clove, minced

- 4 salmon filets

- 4 c. cooked brown rice

- 1 avocado, thinly sliced

- Lime wedges, for serving

Instructions:

1. Preheat oven to 400° and line a large baking sheet with parchment paper. Place bell peppers onto baking sheet and toss with 1 tbsp olive oil. Season with salt and pepper and place in the oven to bake for 10 minutes.

2. Meanwhile, make cilantro lime marinade: combine olive oil, lime juice, cilantro, honey, and garlic and whisk to combine. Place salmon in a large bowl and season with salt and pepper. Pour half the marinade over filets. Toss until fully coated. Set aside remaining marinade.

3. When peppers have baked for 10 minutes, remove from oven and place filets on top of peppers. Bake until peppers are tender and salmon is cooked through, 15 to 20 minutes more.

4. Assemble bowls: divide rice into four bowls and top with salmon, peppers, avocado and a wedge of lime. Garnish with cilantro and serve with extra marinade on the side.

White Bean and Tuna Salad with Basil Vinaigrette

Ingredients:

- Kosher salt

- Pepper

- 12 oz. green beans, trimmed and halved

- 1 small shallot, chopped

- 1 c. lightly packed basil leaves

- 3 tbsp. olive oil

- 1 tbsp. red wine vinegar

- 4 c. oak leaf lettuce or butter lettuce

- 1 15-oz. can small white beans, rinsed

- 2 5-oz. cans solid white tuna in water, drained

- 4 soft- or hard-boiled eggs, halved

Instructions:

1. Bring a large pot of water to a boil. Add 1 tablespoon salt, then green beans, and cook until just tender, 3 to 4 minutes. Drain and rinse under cold water to cool.

2. Meanwhile, in a blender, puree shallot, basil, oil, vinegar, and 1/2 teaspoon each salt and pepper until smooth. Transfer half of dressing to a large bowl and toss with green beans. Fold in lettuce, white beans, and tuna and serve with remaining dressing and eggs.

Moroccan Meatballs with Roasted Tomatoes and Chickpeas

Ingredients:

- 1 large egg

- 1/3 c. panko

- 1 tsp. ground cumin

- 1/4 tsp. ground allspice

- 1/8 tsp. ground cinnamon

- Kosher salt and pepper

- 3 cloves garlic, divided

- 1 lb. ground beef

- 1-pint cherry tomatoes, halved

- 1 14.5-oz can chickpeas, rinsed

- 1 tbsp. olive oil

- 1/4 c. crumbled feta

- 1/4 c. cup fresh flat-leaf parsley, chopped

- Couscous, for serving

Instructions:

1. Heat broiler. In a large bowl, beat egg, then add panko, spices, 1/2 tsp salt, and 1/4 tsp pepper. Finely grate in 2 cloves garlic. Mix in beef, then shape into 12 balls.

2. Transfer meatballs to a rimmed baking sheet, then broil on a rack in the upper portion of the oven until browned, 2 to 3 minutes. Reduce oven temperature to 425°F. Remove meatballs from oven and carefully pour out any excess fat.

3. In a bowl, toss tomatoes and chickpeas with oil, remaining clove garlic (thinly sliced), and 1/4 tsp each salt and pepper. Add to pan with meatballs and roast until tomatoes have softened, about 10 minutes. Remove from oven, top with feta and parsley, and serve with couscous.

Berry Yogurt Parfait

Ingredients:

• 1/2 cup Greek yogurt (low-fat or non-fat)

• 1/4 cup mixed berries (such as strawberries, blueberries, raspberries)

• 2 tablespoons granola (low-sugar or sugar-free)

• 1 tablespoon honey (optional)

Instructions:

1. In a glass or bowl, layer Greek yogurt, mixed berries, and granola. Repeat the layers as desired.

2. Drizzle honey on top for added sweetness if desired.

3. Serve this delightful and protein-rich berry yogurt parfait.

Baked Apples with Cinnamon

Ingredients:

• 2 apples (such as Granny Smith or Honeycrisp), cored and halved

• 1 teaspoon cinnamon

• 1 tablespoon chopped nuts (such as almonds or walnuts)

• 1 tablespoon honey (optional)

Instructions:

1. Preheat the oven to 375°F (190°C).

2. Place the apple halves on a baking dish, cut side up. Sprinkle cinnamon evenly over the apples.

3. Bake for 20-25 minutes or until the apples are tender. Remove from the oven and sprinkle chopped nuts on top.

4. Drizzle honey over the baked apples if desired. Serve these warm and naturally sweet baked apples.

Chia Seed Pudding

Ingredients:

• 2 tablespoons chia seeds

• 1/2 cup unsweetened almond milk (or any preferred milk)

• 1/4 teaspoon vanilla extract

• 1 teaspoon maple syrup or agave syrup (optional)

• Fresh fruit for topping (such as sliced strawberries or blueberries)

Instructions:

1. In a bowl, mix chia seeds, almond milk, vanilla extract, and maple syrup (if using). Stir well.

2. Let the mixture sit for 10 minutes, then stir again to prevent clumping.

3. Cover the bowl and refrigerate for at least 2 hours or overnight until the mixture thickens into a pudding-like consistency.

4. Once set, top the chia seed pudding with fresh fruit before serving.

5. Enjoy this nutritious and fiber-rich chia seed pudding.

Frozen Banana Bites

Ingredients:

- 2 ripe bananas, peeled and sliced

- 1/4 cup unsweetened peanut butter or almond butter

- 1/4 cup dark chocolate chips (at least 70% cocoa)

- 1 tablespoon coconut oil

Instructions:

1. Line a baking sheet with parchment paper.

2. Spread peanut butter or almond butter on one side of each banana slice.

3. Sandwich together to form banana "sandwiches" and place them on the prepared baking sheet.

4. Freeze the banana bites for 1-2 hours until firm.

5. In a microwave-safe bowl, melt dark chocolate chips and coconut oil in 30-second intervals, stirring until smooth.

6. Dip each frozen banana bite halfway into the melted chocolate mixture.

7. Place the coated banana bites back on the parchment paper and freeze for an additional 30 minutes until the chocolate hardens.

8. Enjoy these indulgent yet portion-controlled frozen banana bites.

Yogurt-Covered Berries

Ingredients:

• 1/2 cup Greek yogurt (low-fat or non-fat)

• 1/2 cup mixed berries (such as strawberries, blueberries, raspberries)

Instructions:

1. Dip each berry into Greek yogurt, coating them halfway.

2. Place the yogurt-covered berries on a parchment-lined plate or tray. Freeze for 1-2 hours until the yogurt hardens.

3. Serve these refreshing and protein-packed yogurt-covered berries.

Baked Pear with Cinnamon

Ingredients:

• 2 ripe pears, halved and cored

• 1 teaspoon cinnamon

• 1 tablespoon chopped nuts (such as almonds or pecans)

• 1 tablespoon honey (optional)

Instructions:

1. Preheat the oven to 375°F (190°C).

2. Place the pear halves on a baking dish, cut side up. Sprinkle cinnamon evenly over the pears.

3. Bake for 20-25 minutes or until the pears are tender. Remove from the oven and sprinkle chopped nuts on top.

4. Drizzle honey over the baked pears if desired. Serve these warm and naturally sweet baked pears.

Mini Protein Cheesecake Bites

Ingredients:

• 8 oz cream cheese (low-fat or Greek yogurt cream cheese)

• 1/4 cup plain Greek yogurt

- 1/4 cup protein powder (vanilla or unflavored)

- 2 tablespoons honey or maple syrup

- 1 teaspoon vanilla extract

- Fresh berries for topping (optional)

Instructions:

1. In a mixing bowl, combine cream cheese, Greek yogurt, protein powder, honey or maple syrup, and vanilla extract. Mix until smooth.

2. Line a mini muffin tin with paper liners. Spoon the cheesecake mixture evenly into each muffin cup.

3. Chill in the refrigerator for at least 2 hours or until set.

4. Once set, top each mini cheesecake with fresh berries if desired. Enjoy these protein-packed mini cheesecake bites.

Chocolate Avocado Mousse

Ingredients:

- 2 ripe avocados

- 1/4 cup unsweetened cocoa powder

- 1/4 cup honey or maple syrup

- 1 teaspoon vanilla extract

• Fresh berries for garnish (optional)

Instructions:

1. In a food processor or blender, combine avocados, cocoa powder, honey or maple syrup, and vanilla extract. Blend until smooth and creamy.

2. Divide the chocolate avocado mousse into serving cups or bowls.

3. Chill in the refrigerator for at least 1 hour before serving. Garnish with fresh berries if desired.

4. Serve this rich and creamy chocolate avocado mousse.

Frozen Yogurt Bark

Ingredients:

• 1 cup Greek yogurt (low-fat or non-fat)

• 2 tablespoons honey or maple syrup

• 1/4 cup mixed berries (such as strawberries, blueberries)

• 2 tablespoons chopped nuts (such as almonds or walnuts)

Instructions:

1. Line a baking sheet with parchment paper.

2. In a bowl, mix Greek yogurt and honey or maple syrup until well combined.

3. Spread the yogurt mixture evenly onto the prepared baking sheet. Sprinkle mixed berries and chopped nuts over the yogurt.

4. Freeze for 2-3 hours until the yogurt bark is firm. Break into pieces before serving.

5. Enjoy this refreshing and customizable frozen yogurt bark.

Banana "Ice Cream"

Ingredients:

• 2 ripe bananas, sliced and frozen

• 1/4 cup unsweetened almond milk (or any preferred milk)

• 1 tablespoon unsweetened cocoa powder (optional)

• 1 tablespoon chopped nuts or shredded coconut for topping (optional)

Instructions:

1. Place frozen banana slices in a food processor or blender.

2. Add almond milk and cocoa powder (if using) to the blender. Blend until the mixture reaches a creamy, ice cream-like consistency.

3. Scoop the banana "ice cream" into serving bowls. Top with chopped nuts or shredded coconut if desired.

4. Enjoy this creamy and guilt-free banana "ice cream."

Ingredients:

- 1 cup almond flour

- 2 tablespoons coconut flour

- 1/4 teaspoon baking soda

- Pinch of salt

- 2 tablespoons honey or maple syrup

- 2 tablespoons melted coconut oil

- 2 large eggs

- 1/2 teaspoon vanilla extract

- 1/2 cup fresh blueberries

Instructions:

1. Preheat the oven to 350°F (175°C). Line a muffin tin with paper liners.

2. In a mixing bowl, whisk together almond flour, coconut flour, baking soda, and salt.

3. In another bowl, whisk together honey or maple syrup, melted coconut oil, eggs, and vanilla extract.

4. Combine the wet and dry ingredients until just mixed. Gently fold in the fresh blueberries into the batter.

5. Divide the batter evenly into the muffin cups. Bake for 18-20 minutes or until a toothpick inserted comes out clean.

6. Allow the muffins to cool before serving these delightful almond flour blueberry muffins.

Coconut Chia Seed Pudding with Mango

Ingredients:

• 1/4 cup chia seeds

• 1 cup unsweetened coconut milk

• 1 tablespoon honey or maple syrup

• 1/2 teaspoon vanilla extract

• 1 ripe mango, diced

Instructions:

1. In a bowl, mix chia seeds, coconut milk, honey or maple syrup, and vanilla extract. Stir well.

2. Refrigerate the mixture for at least 2 hours or until it thickens into a pudding-like consistency.

3. Once set, layer the chia seed pudding and diced mango in serving cups.

4. Serve this tropical and satisfying coconut chia seed pudding.

No-Bake Peanut Butter Energy Bites

Ingredients:

- 1 cup rolled oats

- 1/4 cup creamy peanut butter (or any nut/seed butter)

- 1/4 cup honey or maple syrup

- 2 tablespoons ground flaxseed

- 1/4 cup mini dark chocolate chips (optional)

- 1/2 teaspoon vanilla extract

Instructions:

1. In a mixing bowl, combine rolled oats, peanut butter, honey or maple syrup, ground flaxseed, chocolate chips (if using), and vanilla extract.

2. Stir until well combined. Roll the mixture into small bite-sized balls.

3. Place the energy bites on a parchment-lined plate or tray. Refrigerate for at least 30 minutes before serving.

4. Enjoy these convenient and nutritious no-bake peanut butter energy bites.

Ingredients:

• 2 apples (any variety), cored and sliced

• 1 tablespoon melted coconut oil

• 1 teaspoon cinnamon

• 1 tablespoon chopped nuts (such as walnuts or pecans)

• 1 tablespoon honey (optional)

Instructions:

1. Preheat the oven to 350°F (175°C).

2. In a bowl, toss apple slices with melted coconut oil and cinnamon until coated.

3. Arrange the apple slices in a single layer on a baking sheet. Bake for 15-20 minutes or until the apples are tender.

4. Remove from the oven and sprinkle chopped nuts on top. Drizzle honey over the baked apple slices if desired.

5. Serve these warm and aromatic baked cinnamon apple slices.

Pumpkin Pie Chia Seed Pudding

Ingredients:

• 1/4 cup chia seeds

• 1 cup unsweetened almond milk (or any preferred milk)

• 1/4 cup pumpkin puree

• 2 tablespoons maple syrup or honey

• 1/2 teaspoon pumpkin pie spice

• Whipped coconut cream for topping (optional)

Instructions:

1. In a bowl, mix chia seeds, almond milk, pumpkin puree, maple syrup or honey, and pumpkin pie spice. Stir well.

2. Refrigerate the mixture for at least 2 hours or until it thickens into a pudding-like consistency.

3. Once set, spoon the pumpkin pie chia seed pudding into serving cups. Top with whipped coconut cream if desired.

4. Serve this seasonal and flavorful pumpkin pie chia seed pudding.

Avocado Chocolate Pudding

Ingredients:

• 2 ripe avocados

- 1/4 cup unsweetened cocoa powder

- 1/4 cup honey or maple syrup

- 1 teaspoon vanilla extract

- Fresh berries for garnish (optional)

Instructions:

1. Scoop out the avocados and place them in a food processor or blender.

2. Add cocoa powder, honey or maple syrup, and vanilla extract. Blend until the mixture is smooth and creamy.

3. Divide the avocado chocolate pudding into serving bowls. Garnish with fresh berries if desired.

4. Serve this rich and decadent avocado chocolate pudding.

Protein-Packed Banana Bread

Ingredients:

- 2 ripe bananas, mashed

- 2 eggs

- 1/4 cup almond flour

- 1/4 cup vanilla protein powder

- 1/4 teaspoon baking soda

- 1/2 teaspoon cinnamon

- 1/4 cup chopped walnuts or pecans (optional)

Instructions:

1. Preheat the oven to 350°F (175°C). Grease a loaf pan or line it with parchment paper.

2. In a mixing bowl, combine mashed bananas and eggs.

3. Add almond flour, vanilla protein powder, baking soda, cinnamon, and chopped nuts (if using). Mix until well combined.

4. Pour the batter into the prepared loaf pan. Bake for 25-30 minutes or until a toothpick inserted comes out clean.

5. Allow the banana bread to cool before slicing.

6. Enjoy this protein-packed and flavorful banana bread.

Mango Coconut Sorbet

Ingredients:

- 2 ripe mangoes, peeled and diced

- 1 cup unsweetened coconut milk

- 2 tablespoons honey or maple syrup

- 1 tablespoon lime juice

• Shredded coconut for garnish (optional)

Instructions:

1. Place diced mangoes in a blender or food processor.

2. Add coconut milk, honey or maple syrup, and lime juice. Blend until smooth.

3. Pour the mixture into a shallow dish and freeze for 3-4 hours, stirring occasionally for a smooth texture.

4. Scoop the mango coconut sorbet into serving bowls. Garnish with shredded coconut if desired.

5. Serve this refreshing and tropical mango coconut sorbet.

Greek Yogurt Berry Popsicles

Ingredients:

• 1 cup Greek yogurt (low-fat or non-fat)

• 1/2 cup mixed berries (such as strawberries, blueberries)

• 2 tablespoons honey or maple syrup

Instructions:

1. In a bowl, mix Greek yogurt and honey or maple syrup until well combined.

2. Gently fold in the mixed berries. Spoon the mixture into popsicle molds.

3. Insert popsicle sticks and freeze for at least 4 hours or until firm.

4. Run the molds under warm water to release the popsicles before serving.

5. Enjoy these refreshing and protein-rich Greek yogurt berry popsicles.

Cinnamon Baked Peaches

Ingredients:

- 2 ripe peaches, halved and pits removed

- 1 tablespoon melted coconut oil

- 1 teaspoon cinnamon

- 2 tablespoons chopped almonds or pecans

- 1 tablespoon honey (optional)

Instructions:

1. Preheat the oven to 375°F (190°C).

2. Place the peach halves on a baking dish, cut side up. Brush each peach half with melted coconut oil.

3. Sprinkle cinnamon evenly over the peaches. Bake for 20-25 minutes or until the peaches are tender.

4. Remove from the oven and sprinkle chopped nuts on top. Drizzle honey over the baked peaches if desired.

5. Serve these warm and fragrant cinnamon baked peaches.

Ricotta and Berry Parfait

Ingredients:

- 1/2 cup low-fat ricotta cheese

- 1/4 teaspoon vanilla extract

- 1 tablespoon honey or maple syrup

- 1/2 cup mixed berries (such as raspberries, blueberries)

- 1 tablespoon chopped almonds or walnuts

Instructions:

1. In a bowl, mix ricotta cheese, vanilla extract, and honey or maple syrup until smooth.

2. Layer the ricotta mixture and mixed berries in serving glasses or bowls.

3. Sprinkle chopped almonds or walnuts on top.

4. Serve this protein-rich and flavorful ricotta and berry parfait.

Quinoa Banana Cookies

Ingredients:

• 1 cup cooked quinoa, cooled

• 2 ripe bananas, mashed

• 1/4 cup unsweetened applesauce

• 1/4 cup chopped nuts (such as pecans or almonds)

• 1/4 teaspoon cinnamon

• 1/4 teaspoon vanilla extract

Instructions:

1. Preheat the oven to 350°F (175°C). Line a baking sheet with parchment paper.

2. In a bowl, combine cooked quinoa, mashed bananas, applesauce, chopped nuts, cinnamon, and vanilla extract. Mix well.

3. Drop spoonfuls of the mixture onto the prepared baking sheet, shaping them into cookies.

4. Bake for 20-25 minutes or until the edges are golden brown.

5. Allow the quinoa banana cookies to cool before serving.

6. Enjoy these nutritious and naturally sweetened cookies.

Berry Frozen Yogurt Bites

Ingredients:

• 1 cup Greek yogurt (low-fat or non-fat)

• 1/2 cup mixed berries (such as strawberries, blueberries)

• 1 tablespoon honey or maple syrup (optional)

Instructions:

1. In a bowl, mix Greek yogurt and honey or maple syrup until combined. Gently fold in the mixed berries.

2. Spoon the mixture into mini muffin cups or silicone molds. Freeze for 2-3 hours or until firm.

3. Remove the frozen yogurt bites from the molds before serving.

4. Serve these bite-sized and protein-packed berry frozen yogurt bites.

Protein-Packed Pumpkin Pie Bites

Ingredients:

• 1/2 cup pumpkin puree

• 1/4 cup vanilla protein powder

• 2 tablespoons almond flour

• 1 teaspoon pumpkin pie spice

- 1 tablespoon honey or maple syrup (optional)

- Chopped pecans for topping (optional)

Instructions:

1. In a mixing bowl, combine pumpkin puree, vanilla protein powder, almond flour, pumpkin pie spice, and honey or maple syrup (if using). Mix until well combined.

2. Roll the mixture into small bite-sized balls.

3. Optionally, roll the balls in chopped pecans for an added crunch.

4. Place the pumpkin pie bites on a plate or tray. Refrigerate for at least 30 minutes before serving.

5. Enjoy these protein-packed pumpkin pie bites.

Mango Sorbet

Ingredients:

- 2 ripe mangoes, peeled and diced

- 2 tablespoons honey or maple syrup

- 1 tablespoon lime juice

- Fresh mint leaves for garnish (optional)

Instructions:

1. Place diced mangoes in a blender or food processor.

2. Add honey or maple syrup and lime juice. Blend until smooth.

3. Transfer the mango mixture into a shallow dish and freeze for 3-4 hours, stirring occasionally for a smooth texture.

4. Scoop the mango sorbet into serving bowls. Garnish with fresh mint leaves if desired.

5. Serve this refreshing and naturally sweet mango sorbet.

Apple Cinnamon Baked Oatmeal Cups

Ingredients:

• 1 cup rolled oats

• 1/4 teaspoon baking powder

• 1 teaspoon cinnamon

• 1/4 cup unsweetened applesauce

• 1/4 cup almond milk (or any preferred milk)

• 1 small apple, diced

• 1 tablespoon honey or maple syrup

• Chopped nuts for topping (optional)

Instructions:

1. Preheat the oven to 350°F (175°C). Grease a muffin tin or line it with liners.

2. In a bowl, mix rolled oats, baking powder, and cinnamon.

3. Add applesauce, almond milk, diced apple, and honey or maple syrup. Stir until combined.

4. Spoon the mixture into the prepared muffin cups, filling each about 3/4 full. Sprinkle chopped nuts on top if desired.

5. Bake for 20-25 minutes or until the tops are golden brown and set.

6. Allow the oatmeal cups to cool before removing from the tin.

7. Serve these individual-sized and fiber-rich apple cinnamon baked oatmeal cups.

Chocolate Banana Protein Smoothie

Ingredients:

• 1 ripe banana

• 1 cup unsweetened almond milk (or any preferred milk)

• 1 scoop chocolate protein powder

• 1 tablespoon unsweetened cocoa powder

• 1 tablespoon almond butter or peanut butter

• Ice cubes (optional)

Instructions:

1. Place all the ingredients in a blender. Blend until smooth and creamy.

2. Add ice cubes if a colder consistency is desired.

3. Pour into a glass and serve this protein-rich and indulgent chocolate banana smoothie.

Blueberry Chia Seed Jam

Ingredients:

• 1 cup fresh or frozen blueberries

• 2 tablespoons chia seeds

• 1-2 tablespoons honey or maple syrup (optional)

• 1 teaspoon lemon juice

Instructions:

1. In a saucepan, heat the blueberries over medium heat, stirring occasionally until they start to break down.

2. Mash the blueberries with a fork or potato masher.

3. Add chia seeds, honey or maple syrup (if using), and lemon juice. Stir well. Simmer for 5-7 minutes until the mixture thickens.

4. Remove from heat and let it cool. The jam will thicken further as it cools.

5. Transfer to a jar or container and refrigerate.

6. Serve this homemade and naturally sweetened blueberry chia seed jam.

Cinnamon Roasted Almonds

Ingredients:

- 1 cup raw almonds

- 1 tablespoon melted coconut oil

- 1 tablespoon honey or maple syrup

- 1 teaspoon cinnamon

- Pinch of salt

Instructions:

1. Preheat the oven to 300°F (150°C). Line a baking sheet with parchment paper.

2. In a bowl, mix raw almonds, melted coconut oil, honey or maple syrup, cinnamon, and salt until the almonds are evenly coated.

3. Spread the almonds in a single layer on the prepared baking sheet.

4. Bake for 20-25 minutes, stirring occasionally, until the almonds are toasted and fragrant.

5. Remove from the oven and let them cool completely.

6. Serve these aromatic and lightly sweetened cinnamon roasted almonds as a snack.

Lemon Ricotta Poppy Seed Muffins

Ingredients:

• 1 cup almond flour

• 2 tablespoons coconut flour

• 1/4 teaspoon baking soda

• Pinch of salt

• 2 tablespoons poppy seeds

• Zest of 1 lemon

• 1/4 cup low-fat ricotta cheese

• 2 tablespoons melted coconut oil

• 2 tablespoons honey or maple syrup

• 2 large eggs

• 1 tablespoon lemon juice

Instructions:

1. Preheat the oven to 350°F (175°C). Grease a muffin tin or use liners.

2. In a bowl, mix almond flour, coconut flour, baking soda, salt, poppy seeds, and lemon zest.

3. In another bowl, combine ricotta cheese, melted coconut oil, honey or maple syrup, eggs, and lemon juice. Mix well.

4. Gradually add the dry ingredients to the wet ingredients and stir until combined.

5. Spoon the batter into the muffin cups, filling each about 3/4 full. Bake for 18-20 minutes or until a toothpick inserted comes out clean.

6. Allow the muffins to cool before serving these delightful lemon ricotta poppy seed muffins.

Veggie Sticks with Hummus

Ingredients:

- Assorted vegetables (carrots, cucumber, bell peppers)

- 1/2 cup homemade or store-bought hummus

Instructions:

1. Wash and cut assorted vegetables into sticks.

2. Arrange the vegetable sticks on a plate or in a bento box. Serve with a side of hummus for dipping.

3. Enjoy this crunchy and nutritious snack.

Turkey and Cheese Roll-Ups

Ingredients:

- 4 slices of deli turkey or chicken

- 2 slices of low-fat cheese (cheddar, Swiss)

- Mustard or low-fat mayo (optional)

- Lettuce leaves

Instructions:

1. Lay the turkey slices flat. Place a slice of cheese on top of each turkey slice.

2. Optionally, spread mustard or low-fat mayo on the cheese. Add a lettuce leaf on top.

3. Roll up the turkey slices with cheese and lettuce. Secure with a toothpick if needed.

4. Serve these protein-packed turkey and cheese roll-ups.

Greek Yogurt and Berry Parfait

Ingredients:

- 1/2 cup Greek yogurt (low-fat or non-fat)

- 1/4 cup mixed berries (strawberries, blueberries)

- 1 tablespoon chopped nuts or granola (optional)

- 1 teaspoon honey or maple syrup (optional)

Instructions:

1. In a glass or small bowl, layer Greek yogurt and mixed berries. Repeat the layers as desired.

2. Sprinkle chopped nuts or granola on top if using. Drizzle honey or maple syrup for added sweetness if desired.

3. Serve this protein-rich and antioxidant-packed parfait.

Cottage Cheese and Pineapple Cups

Ingredients:

- 1/2 cup low-fat cottage cheese

- 1/2 cup diced pineapple (fresh or canned in juice)

- Mint leaves for garnish (optional)

Instructions:

1. Divide the cottage cheese into serving cups.

2. Top each cup with diced pineapple. Garnish with mint leaves if desired.

3. Serve these simple and protein-filled cottage cheese and pineapple cups.

Baked Kale Chips

Ingredients:

- 1 bunch of kale, washed and dried

- 1 tablespoon olive oil

- Salt and pepper to taste

Instructions:

1. Preheat the oven to 300°F (150°C). Line a baking sheet with parchment paper.

2. Remove the kale leaves from the stems and tear into bite-sized pieces.

3. In a bowl, toss kale pieces with olive oil, salt, and pepper until coated. Spread the kale pieces in a single layer on the prepared baking sheet.

4. Bake for 10-15 minutes until the kale is crispy but not burnt. Remove from the oven and let them cool completely.

5. Serve these crunchy and nutrient-packed baked kale chips.

Peanut Butter Banana Bites

Ingredients:

• 1 ripe banana, sliced

• 2 tablespoons natural peanut butter (or any nut/seed butter)

• 2 tablespoons chopped nuts (such as almonds or walnuts)

Instructions:

1. Spread each banana slice with a thin layer of peanut butter.

2. Sprinkle chopped nuts on top of the peanut butter. Arrange the peanut butter-covered banana slices on a plate.

3. Serve these simple and satisfying peanut butter banana bites.

Egg Salad Cucumber Bites

Ingredients:

• 2 hard-boiled eggs, peeled and chopped

- 2 tablespoons Greek yogurt

- 1 teaspoon mustard

- Salt and pepper to taste

- 1 large cucumber, sliced into rounds

Instructions:

1. In a bowl, mix chopped hard-boiled eggs, Greek yogurt, mustard, salt, and pepper until well combined.

2. Place a spoonful of egg salad onto each cucumber round.

3. Serve these protein-packed and refreshing egg salad cucumber bites.

Rice Cake with Avocado and Tomato

Ingredients:

- 1 rice cake (plain or multigrain)

- 1/4 ripe avocado, mashed

- 1 small tomato, sliced

- Sprinkle of salt and pepper (optional)

Instructions:

1. Spread mashed avocado evenly onto the rice cake. Top with tomato slices.

2. Add a sprinkle of salt and pepper if desired.

3. Serve this simple and healthy rice cake with avocado and tomato.

Cottage Cheese and Berries Bowl

Ingredients:

- 1/2 cup low-fat cottage cheese

- 1/2 cup mixed berries (such as raspberries, blackberries)

- 1 tablespoon chopped nuts or seeds

Instructions:

1. In a bowl, spoon the cottage cheese.

2. Top with mixed berries and chopped nuts or seeds.

3. Serve this protein-rich and antioxidant-filled cottage cheese and berries bowl.

Veggie and Hummus Snack Box

Ingredients:

- Assorted vegetable sticks (carrots, celery, bell peppers)

- 1/4 cup hummus

- 2 tablespoons nuts or seeds (almonds, pumpkin seeds)

Instructions:

1. Arrange assorted vegetable sticks in a compartment of a snack box or plate.

2. Add a portion of hummus in a separate compartment. Place nuts or seeds in another compartment.

3. Serve this balanced and satisfying veggie and hummus snack box.

Caprese Skewers

Ingredients:

• Cherry tomatoes

• Fresh mozzarella cheese balls

• Fresh basil leaves

• Balsamic glaze (optional)

Instructions:

1. Thread cherry tomatoes, mozzarella cheese balls, and fresh basil leaves onto small skewers or toothpicks.

2. Drizzle with balsamic glaze if desired.

3. Serve these flavorful and portion-controlled Caprese skewers.

Tuna Cucumber Boats

Ingredients:

- 1 can (5 oz) tuna, drained

- 2 tablespoons Greek yogurt

- 1 teaspoon Dijon mustard

- 1 small cucumber, cut into halves lengthwise

- Chopped fresh herbs (such as parsley or dill)

- Salt and pepper to taste

Instructions:

1. In a bowl, mix tuna, Greek yogurt, Dijon mustard, chopped herbs, salt, and pepper until combined.

2. Scoop out the seeds from the cucumber halves to form "boats."

3. Fill each cucumber boat with the tuna mixture.

4. Serve these protein-packed and refreshing tuna cucumber boats.

Roasted Chickpeas

Ingredients:

- 1 can (15 oz) chickpeas, drained and rinsed

- 1 tablespoon olive oil

- 1 teaspoon smoked paprika

- 1/2 teaspoon garlic powder

- 1/2 teaspoon cumin

- Salt to taste

Instructions:

1. Preheat the oven to 400°F (200°C). Line a baking sheet with parchment paper.

2. Pat dry the chickpeas with a paper towel to remove excess moisture.

3. In a bowl, toss chickpeas with olive oil, smoked paprika, garlic powder, cumin, and salt until coated.

4. Spread the chickpeas in a single layer on the prepared baking sheet. Roast for 25-30 minutes or until crispy, shaking the pan occasionally.

5. Remove from the oven and let them cool completely. Serve these crunchy and fiber-rich roasted chickpeas.

Apple Sandwiches with Almond Butter

Ingredients:

• 1 apple, cored and sliced horizontally

• 2 tablespoons almond butter (or any nut/seed butter)

• Unsweetened coconut flakes (optional)

• Mini chocolate chips (optional)

Instructions:

1. Spread almond butter on one side of each apple slice.

2. Optionally, sprinkle unsweetened coconut flakes or mini chocolate chips on the almond butter.

3. Place another apple slice on top to form a "sandwich."

4. Serve these delicious and fiber-filled apple sandwiches.

Edamame Snack Bowl

Ingredients:

• 1 cup edamame (shelled)

• 1 teaspoon sesame oil

• 1/2 teaspoon sesame seeds

• Pinch of chili flakes (optional)

• Pinch of sea salt

Instructions:

1. Bring a pot of water to a boil and blanch the edamame for 3-4 minutes.

2. Drain and pat dry the edamame.

3. Toss the edamame with sesame oil, sesame seeds, chili flakes (if using), and sea salt.

4. Serve this protein-packed and flavorful edamame snack bowl.

CONCLUSION

The decision to undergo gastric bypass surgery marks the beginning of a transformative journey toward a healthier lifestyle. This surgical intervention, although significant, is merely a stepping stone towards a life of improved well-being. It signifies not just a physical change but a commitment to embracing a new relationship with food, exercise, and overall self-care.

Gastric bypass surgery is a tool that assists in weight loss by altering the anatomy of the digestive system. However, its success is profoundly influenced by the patient's dedication to making sustainable lifestyle adjustments. Post-surgery, individuals must adapt to a new way of eating, prioritizing nutrition, portion control, and mindful choices. Exercise becomes a crucial component, fostering not only physical strength but also mental resilience.

While the surgery offers profound benefits in terms of weight loss, improved health markers, and increased mobility, its true success lies in the long-term commitment to maintaining these positive changes. The journey after surgery encompasses ongoing support, making informed dietary choices, establishing consistent exercise routines, and nurturing mental and emotional well-being.

It's imperative to recognize that gastric bypass surgery is not a quick fix but a tool that empowers individuals to take charge of their health. Each step taken post-surgery, every meal planned mindfully, every physical activity embraced, and every moment of self-reflection contributes to a healthier and more fulfilling life.

Ultimately, the conclusion of the gastric bypass surgery journey is not the end but the beginning of a lifelong commitment to health, wellness, and a renewed sense of vitality. It's about celebrating achievements, embracing challenges, and creating a future filled with well-being, balance, and sustained vitality. With dedication, perseverance, and support, individuals can truly thrive and lead a fulfilling life beyond the confines of their initial health concerns.